Independent Prescribing for District Nursing

Edited by

Amanda Blaber, Hannah Ingram and Jennifer Gorman

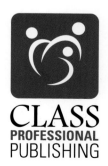

CLASS
PROFESSIONAL
PUBLISHING

Printing history
This edition first published 2020

The authors and publisher welcome feedback from the users of this book. Please contact the publisher:

Class Professional Publishing,
The Exchange, Express Park, Bristol Road, Bridgwater TA6 4RR
Telephone: 01278 472 800
Email: post@class.co.uk
Website: www.classprofessional.co.uk

Class Professional Publishing is an imprint of Class Publishing Ltd

A CIP catalogue record for this book is available from the British Library

Paperback ISBN: 9781859598627
eBook ISBN: 9781859598610

Cover design by Hybert Design Limited, UK
Designed and typeset by S4Carlisle Publishing Services
Printed in the UK by Short Run Press

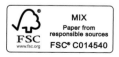

Contents

Disclaimer

The details in this book are presented for information purposes only. Healthcare professionals should be aware of their own scope of practice and rely on their own experience and knowledge in evaluating and using any information, methods, or compounds described herein. In light of rapid advances in medical science, independent verifications of diagnoses and drug dosages should be made. To the fullest extent of the law, no responsibility is assumed by the publishers or authors, for any injury and/or damage to persons or property as a matter of products liability, negligence or otherwise, or from any use or operation of any methods, products, instructions or ideas described herein.

About the Authors

Editors

Amanda Blaber

Amanda has 17 years teaching experience in higher education institutes, with many years of emergency care experience. Amanda contributes to the Forum for Higher Education for Paramedics and the Council of Deans Paramedic Advisory group. Amanda is an Honorary Fellow of the College of Paramedics and is extremely proud of the literary contribution she and her colleagues have made to the education of paramedics in the UK. Amanda has extensive knowledge and experience in curriculum design and validation processes and is a Senior Fellow of the Higher Education Academy. As a lecturer, Amanda finds inspiration and enjoyment from teaching and endeavours to make students' learning as real and as fun as possible. Amanda has published (alone and with colleagues) four paramedic texts, two of which are bestsellers and have resulted in further editions being written. Amanda is committed to supporting early career writers to have the opportunity to develop their skills and experience in the publishing arena. Amanda has been educated about 'prescribing' from her fellow editors during this process and has enjoyed learning much more about this fascinating area of practice.

Hannah Ingram

Hannah had extensive experience as a district nurse and an advanced nurse practitioner in primary care before commencing her academic career four years ago. Hannah is a principal lecturer and programme lead for independent prescribing in health sciences. She has 13 years prescribing practice experience and enjoys being able to facilitate others to undertake safe and effective prescribing practice within a variety of clinical and professional roles.

Hannah has published in the field of district nursing and recognises the challenges faced by practitioners working in primary care settings and lone roles in the context of prescribing. Hannah has worked particularly with older people and in long-term condition management in her nursing practice, and has successfully facilitated a range of multidisciplinary healthcare practitioners to successfully complete the independent prescribing programme.

Jennifer Gorman

Jennifer is a pharmacist with over 15 years experience. Her career has involved working with a wide range of patient groups in a variety of care settings, including community pharmacy, hospital pharmacy and general practice. She has also worked as a pharmaceutical advisor for a CCG supporting local commissioning. In more recent years she has moved into various academic positions teaching medical students, pharmacists, nurses and paramedics. Currently she is a Senior Lecturer in Pharmacy Practice at the University of Brighton.

Contributor

Vicky Donno is an independent prescriber and advanced nurse practitioner in general practice, with a background in district nursing and primary care. Vicky also holds the PGCert in health and social care education and contributes to the teaching, learning and assessment of the independent prescribing programme at the University of Brighton.

Acknowledgements

The authors would like to thank the following for their input:

- Vicky Donno, Mike Ellis-Martin, Dr Stewart Glaspole, Louise Hatcher and Dr Sian Williams for their expertise and invaluable feedback on the text.
- Samantha Soanes – for support and feedback as a critical friend in the development of the text and contribution towards the case studies.
- All colleagues within the School of Health Sciences and the School of Pharmacy at Brighton University for their invaluable support and constructive feedback as well as colleagues working locally within the NHS who have provided such useful advice.

List of Abbreviations and Acronyms

AACE	Association of Ambulance Chief Executives
ACE	angiotensin-converting enzyme
ADME	absorption, distribution, metabolism and elimination
ADRs	adverse drug reactions
AGS	American Geriatrics Society
AKI	acute kidney injury
APC	Area Prescribing Committee
ARB	angiotensin II receptor antagonist
ARR	absolute risk reduction
AUC	area under the curve
BNF	British National Formulary
BTS	British Thoracic Society
CAS	central alerting system
CASP	Critical Appraisal Skills Programme
CCG	Clinical Commissioning Group
CD	controlled drug
CHD	coronary heart disease
CI	confidence interval
CKD	chronic kidney disease
CKS	Clinical Knowledge Summary
CMP	clinical management plan
CNS	central nervous system
CoP	College of Paramedics
COPD	chronic obstructive pulmonary disease
COX	cyclooxygenase
CPD	continuing professional development
CrCl	creatinine clearance
CVD	cardiovascular disease
DHSS	Department of Health and Social Security
DKA	diabetic ketoacidosis
DoH	Department of Health
DVT	deep vein thrombosis

eGFR	estimated glomerular filtration rate
ePACT	electronic Prescribing Analysis and Cost Tool
GDPR	General Data Protection Regulation
GFR	glomerular filtration rate
GI	gastrointestinal
GMC	General Medical Council
GPCRs	G-protein coupled receptors
GPhC	General Pharmaceutical Council
GSL	general sales list
HAIs	hospital-acquired infections
HCPC	Health and Care Professions Council
HIV	Human Immunodeficiency Virus
HMR	Human Medicines Regulations
ICE	ideas, concerns and expectations
ICER	incremental cost-effectiveness ratio
ICS	inhaled corticosteroids
IM	intramuscular
INR	Internationalised Normalised Ratio
IPDAS	International Patient Decision Aid Standards
IV	intravenous
JVP	jugular venous pressure
LABA	long-acting bronchodilator
LAMA	long-acting antimuscarinic antagonist
LFT	liver function test
MAR	Medicines Administration Record
MDI	metered dose inhaler
MDT	multidisciplinary team
MECC	Making Every Contact Count
MHRA	Medicines and Healthcare products Regulatory Agency
MI	myocardial infarction
MI	motivational interviewing
MRSA	methicillin-resistant Staphylococcus aureus
NHS	National Health Service
NHSBSA	NHS Business Services Authority
NICE	National Institute of Health and Care Excellence
NMC	Nursing and Midwifery Council
NMP	non-medical prescribing

NMS	New Medicines Service
NNT	number needed to treat
NOAC	new oral anti-coagulant
NPC	National Prescribing Centre
NPF	Nurse Prescribers' Formulary
NRLS	National Reporting and Learning System
NRT	nicotine replacement therapy
NSAID	non-steroidal anti-inflammatory drug
OPAT	outpatient parenteral antibiotic therapy
OTC	over the counter
PCD	person-centred development
PEG	percutaneous endoscopic gastroscopy
PGD	Patient Group Direction
PHE	Public Health England
PHOF	Public Health Outcomes Framework
PIM	potentially inappropriate medicine
POM	prescription only medicine
PRN	*pro re nata* (as required)
PSD	Patient Specific Direction
PSRB	Professional Statutory Regulatory Body
QALY	quality-adjusted life year
QDS	*quarter die sumendus* (four times a day)
RA	rheumatoid arthritis
RCGP	Royal College of General Physicians
RCN	Royal College of Nursing
RCT	randomised controlled trial
RPS	Royal Pharmaceutical Society
RRR	relative risk reduction
SABA	short-acting bronchodilator
SAMA	short-acting muscarinic antagonist
SC	subcutaneous
SCR	Summary Care Record
SDM	shared decision-making
SGLT2	sodium-glucose cotransporter 2 inhibitor
SIGN	Scottish Intercollegiate Guidelines Network
SPC	Summary of Product Characteristics
SPS	Specialist Pharmacy Services

SSRI	selective serotonin reuptake inhibitor
SWOT	strengths, weaknesses, opportunities and threats
TA	technology appraisal
TDM	therapeutic drug monitoring
U&Es	urea & electrolytes
UTI	urinary tract infection
Vd	volume of distribution
WHO	World Health Organization

Chapter 1

Background to Prescribing for District Nurses

Hannah Ingram

In This Chapter

♦ Introduction
♦ Prescribing
♦ Prescriber annotation
♦ Social prescribing
♦ History of prescribing by nurses
♦ History of non-medical prescribing
♦ Barriers to independent district nurse prescribing
♦ Impact and benefits of independent district nurse prescribing
♦ Conclusion
♦ Key points of this chapter
♦ References and further reading.

Introduction

This chapter aims to provide a brief overview and an understanding of the evolution of nurse prescribing and independent prescribing in the UK context of healthcare. The differing contexts of prescribing will be considered, as will social prescribing.

Prescribing

Prescribing is to provide an authorisation, be it an appliance, equipment or a drug, for a patient for a specific condition or reason based on a clinical assessment. This requires the prescriber to be legally accountable for the act of their decision making in prescribing; thus, to prescribe requires competence, knowledge and skill in the clinical area and professional specialism in which you are prescribing. As an NMC registrant, you are also accountable for any omissions in care and this extends to prescribing practice once you are annotated as an independent prescriber on the NMC register.

In UK law, only appropriate practitioners can prescribe medicines, a prescriber being a healthcare professional who can write a prescription (NHS UK 2017).

The traditional context of prescribing in the UK has been that of doctors prescribing, pharmacists dispensing and nurses administering (Clegg 2001); however, in contemporary healthcare contexts, this has evolved over the years.

There is a plethora of terms for prescribers that have developed since the initiation of prescribing by practitioners other than medics, and this can cause confusion. Terms such as nurse prescriber, non-medical prescriber, independent prescriber, supplementary prescriber, extended scope prescriber, health visitor prescriber and community nurse prescriber have all been used, sometimes interchangeably, and this chapter aims to set out the correct use and terms of each annotation of prescriber.

Currently in UK law, there are a number of appropriate practitioners who are able to authorise and write prescriptions from different formularies, having completed and passed a Professional and Statutory Body-regulated university course (NHS UK 2017).

Prescriber Annotation

Once the university Professional Statutory Regulatory Body (PSRB) programme has been completed and successfully passed, practitioners can annotate themselves as prescribers with their regulatory body. For nurses this is the Nursing and Midwifery Council (NMC) and for allied health professionals the Health Care Professions Council (HCPC); for doctors and dentists it is the General Medical Council (GMC) and for pharmacists the General Pharmaceutical Council (GPhC).

Prescribing annotations registerable in the UK include:

Community Practitioner Nurse Prescribers

Community nurse prescribers with a specialist practice qualification (SPQ) (such as the community specialist practice award of district nursing) are able to prescribe from the Nurse Prescribers' Formulary if they have undertaken and successfully completed the NMC-regulated V100 prescribing programme and their SPQ award.

Community nurses without a specialist practice qualification can prescribe from the Nurse Prescribers' Formulary if they have undertaken and successfully completed the NMC-regulated V150 prescribing programme (BNF 2019).

A range of *non-medical* prescribers can prescribe medicines for patients as either supplementary or independent prescribers.

Independent Prescribers

Independent prescribers are responsible and accountable for the assessment of patients with undiagnosed or diagnosed conditions, and for decisions regarding their clinical management, which includes prescribing (BNF 2019).

Non-medical or independent prescribers can be:

♦ Dentists
♦ Doctors
♦ Nurses/midwives
♦ Optometrists
♦ Paramedics
♦ Pharmacists
♦ Physiotherapists
♦ Podiatrists
♦ Therapeutic radiologists.

Supplementary Prescribers

Supplementary prescribing refers to a partnership between an independent prescriber (who must be a doctor or a dentist in the context of supplementary prescribing) and a supplementary prescriber to implement an agreed clinical management plan for a specific patient and a specific condition using agreed and specific medications (BNF 2019).

Supplementary prescribers can be (NHS 2017):

♦ Dietitians
♦ Diagnostic and therapeutic radiologists
♦ Nurses/midwives
♦ Optometrists
♦ Paramedics
♦ Pharmacists
♦ Physiotherapists
♦ Podiatrists.

Further information on these prescribing annotations can be found in **Chapter 9**.

As a prescriber, you may have more than one prescribing annotation. See **Case Study 1.1** for an example.

Some people may also be dual registered, for example as a paramedic and as a nurse; however, you must only use your prescribing with the Professional, Statutory and Regulatory body you are registered with, for example the NMC, and who you are employed by, where prescribing is a recognised part of your job role. You must also only use your prescribing where you have liability insurance, it is part of your job description and you have your employer's support to do so.

Case Study 1.1

Sue obtained her specialist practice qualification in district nursing. As part of this she completed the V100, prescribing from the community nurse prescribers' formulary for nurses with a SPQ. Sue registered as a district nurse and was prescribing in practice from the Nurse Prescribers' Formulary (NPF), regularly prescribing dressings, emollients and appliances for her patients.

As Sue developed her skills, knowledge and experience in district nursing specialist practice, she identified that prescribing from a wider formulary would benefit her patients, as she needed to prescribe a wider range of medicines to ensure timely access to treatment. Sue identified that antibiotics, topical steroids and palliative care medications would be within her scope of practice. She discussed this with her line manager and non-medical prescribing lead, and went on to undertake and successfully complete the V300 independent prescribers' course.

The following year, Sue identified that she was nursing more within long-term conditions in her specialist district nursing role, caring for patients with diabetes, COPD and heart failure on a more regular basis. She discussed with her line manager and non-medical prescribing lead that it would be of benefit for her to be able to prescribe within these areas, but that this was currently outside of her scope of prescribing practice. As part of her continuing professional development (CPD) and prescribing development, Sue undertook some further education in these areas and worked collaboratively with one of the GPs in her local area to develop her skills and knowledge in these clinical areas. As she had qualified as an independent prescriber, this also enabled her to undertake supplementary prescribing as part of this annotation. Therefore, Sue undertook supplementary prescribing in these disease areas, prescribing specific medications for specific patients using a clinical management plan in partnership with the GP and with the patients' consent. This aided her in building her competence and confidence in adding further medicines to her scope of prescribing practice.

Had Sue qualified as a supplementary prescriber, this would not have allowed her to undertake independent prescribing. Independent prescribing incorporates supplementary prescribing, but not the other way around.

Social Prescribing

Social prescribing has often been referred to as a community referral. Social prescribing allows district nurses and other healthcare practitioners to refer to local community services, often non-clinical services, to improve physical and mental health and wellbeing (King's Fund 2017).

Social prescribing is not a new concept; it was highlighted in the White Paper *Our Health, Our Care, Our Say* (DoH 2006) as a way to promote health and independence. It was revisited in the NHS *Five Year Forward View* (NHS England 2014) to focus on proactive approaches to wellbeing and patient care. The *General Practice Forward View* (NHS England 2016b) also advocates for social prescribing to reduce pressure on GP services and primary care (King's Fund 2017).

Undertaking social prescribing does not require an NMC qualification as community nurse prescribing, independent prescribing and supplementary prescribing do. Social prescribing may complement your prescribing practice as you refer your patients to other clinical and non-clinical services and third-sector services as available and appropriate.

Social prescribing has been developed since its initial appearance in the government's White Paper (DoH 2006). NHS England now promotes a link worker for agencies to refer their patients and clients to, and the link worker will be able to provide time for the person to focus on what is important for them and facilitate a holistic approach to meeting health and wellbeing needs. Social prescribing will be of benefit to those patients with long-term multiple comorbidities, mental health needs, complex social needs or who are socially isolated (NHS 2019).

As a district nurse, you will be well versed in caring for such patient groups and will be facilitating social prescribing in your practice, even if there is not a standard model of social prescribing in place in your area. As you develop as an independent prescriber, it is important to recognise how your prescribing decisions may impact on the social aspects of a person's life, and how social prescribing and personalised patient-centred care may complement your prescribing decisions for positive health and social outcomes.

History of Prescribing by Nurses

We will now explore how prescribing for nurses developed in healthcare in the UK, and in doing so will begin to understand and recognise how other prescribing names and titles have developed, evolved and become obsolete, as prescribing practice has developed and become part of everyday practice for non-medical healthcare practitioners, and in particular for district nurses.

Non-medical prescribing refers to prescribing practice that is undertaken by a healthcare practitioner without a medical background. Nurses were the first professional group to undertake non-medical prescribing practice in the UK. Nurse prescribing in the UK has its roots in community and district nursing practice.

Baroness Julia Cumberlege, a politician, issued a report in 1986 recommending that community nurses be able to prescribe from a limited list of drugs and appliances (RCN 2014). Her report, *Neighbourhood Nursing: A Focus for Care* (The Cumberlege Report) (DHSS 1986), explored the care that was received by patients from district nurses and health visitors. The report highlighted that district nurses and health visitors were wasting valuable nursing time requesting and obtaining dressings, emollients and appliances from patients' GPs, and that this often resulted in complex prescribing procedures (Courtenay and Griffiths 2010). Baroness Cumberlege reported that care, treatment and patient experience could be enhanced if district nurses and health visitors could prescribe (Cope et al. 2016).

Following the Cumberlege Report (DHSS 1986), the recommendations were reviewed by an advisory group for the Department of Health examining nurse prescribing, led by Dr June Crown in 1989. The Crown Report (DoH 1989) highlighted the complex prescribing patterns that were occurring in practice, with GPs prescribing for patients based on a district nurse's assessment and advice, and time being wasted for patients and staff. Therefore, Dr June Crown ascertained that government action was required to develop prescribing practice and professional responsibility for nurses. The Crown Report identified that suitably qualified community nurses should be able to prescribe from a limited list and to adjust medications within a protocol, and both within clearly defined circumstances (DoH 1989). Patients who were identified as benefiting from nurse prescribing were those with continence needs or wound care and homeless communities not registered with a GP. Another perceived advantage of nurse prescribing was improved communication in primary care teams, where the boundaries of responsibility in prescribing practice would be more clearly and definitively defined (Courtenay and Griffiths 2010).

Despite this, it was a further three years until legislation was changed in 1992 (*Medicinal Products: Prescription by Nurses and Others Act*, DoH 1992), allowing district nurses and health visitors to prescribe from a limited list within the restrictions set out by the Crown Report (DoH 1989). However, the secondary legislation that was needed in order for this practice to be implemented was not amended and passed in this Act until 1994 (University of Stirling 2006). Following the amended Act in 1994, eight pilot sites were set up in England for nurse prescribing from a limited list (Courtenay and Griffiths 2010). Following the success of this pilot programme, the Department of Health introduced prescribing by district nurses and health visitors nationally from 1996. The Nurse Prescribers' Formulary for District Nurses and Health Visitors was the limited list that enabled community nurses' prescribers to prescribe from a range of dressings, medicines, appliances and emollients (University of Stirling 2006). The legislation was updated further in 2005 and 2007, allowing any community nurse (including those without a specialist practice district nurse or health visitor qualification) to prescribe from this formulary on completion of the regulated educational programme. This nurses' formulary had a name change in 2005 to the Nurse Prescribers' Formulary, which remains the current formulary for this group of prescribers whose annotation with the NMC is Community Practitioner Nurse Prescriber with either the V100 or V150 qualification.

A second report by Dr June Crown (DoH 1999b) reviewed the prescribing by nurses and evaluated the research evidence base that had evolved since it was initiated in 1996. Initial research evidence was positive for nurse prescribing. It found that (Luker et al. 1997, 1998):

♦ Patients were satisfied
♦ Time was utilised more efficiently
♦ Patients received treatments more efficiently
♦ Nurses were able to provide better information to their patients regarding treatment
♦ Nurses felt increased satisfaction, autonomy and sense of status.

Based on this evidence, in her second report Dr Crown advocated for it to be a practice that could be adopted by healthcare professionals other than doctors and dentists, district nurses and health visitors, who had specialist expertise and prescribing education. The second Crown Report also recommended further additions to the formulary for nurse prescribers.

Concurrent with Dr Crown's second report, the Department of Health published *Making a Difference* (DoH 1999a) and the *NHS Plan, a Plan for Investment, a Plan for Reform* (DoH 2001b). These government policies were focused on developing the roles and practice scope of nurses, including making it easier for them to prescribe to provide services that were developed and designed around patients, and that ensured patients received a more timely and convenient service (University of Stirling 2006).

The nurse prescribing formulary was subsequently extended by the government in 2001, when funding was given for qualified nurse prescribers and nurses new to prescribing to undertake training to prescribe from the Nurse Prescribers' Extended Formulary, annotated by the NMC as V200 prescribers. This extended formulary included some prescription-only medicines, some general sales list medicines and some pharmacy-only medicines. This formulary had numerous additions to the list between 2003 and 2006 (Courtenay and Griffiths 2010).

History of Non-medical Prescribing

In 2003, the government developed prescribing for non-medical practitioners further. This was through the introduction of supplementary prescribing for nurses and pharmacists. Supplementary prescribing is defined as the voluntary agreement between the independent prescriber – a doctor or a dentist – and the supplementary prescriber to implement an agreed patient-specific clinical management plan with the patient's agreement (NMC 2006). Section 63 of the Health and Social Care Act (DoH 2001a) allowed the government to extend supplementary prescribing rights to other healthcare professionals to allow for prescribing by attaching conditions to their prescribing practice, and subsequently optometrists, physiotherapists and podiatrists were able to become supplementary prescribers following further legislative changes in 2005 (DoH 2005a).

In 2006 legislation was passed (DoH 2005b) allowing nurses to independently prescribe any licensed medication for any condition within their scope of practice and sphere of competence, including some controlled drugs. This led to the withdrawal of the V200 annotation and of extended formulary nurse prescribers. Nurse prescribers then became community practitioner nurse prescribers or independent nurse prescribers, depending on their qualification and scope of practice (NMC 2006).

In 2009, further legislation extended independent prescribing for nurses to include unlicensed medications and to mix medicines themselves or direct others to (MHRA 2009), and from April 2012 further changes were made allowing nurse independent prescribers to prescribe virtually any controlled drugs within their competence. This also extended to mixing and giving directions for mixing of controlled drugs (RCN 2014), which is essential for delivering palliative care in the home for district nurses.

Independent prescribing status was extended to pharmacists in 2006 (DoH 2005b). Optometrists were made eligible to become independent prescribers in 2007 (DoH 2007), followed by physiotherapists and podiatrists in 2013 (DoH 2013). In 2016 the NHS announced legislation allowing for independent prescribing for therapeutic radiographers and supplementary prescribing for dieticians. Paramedics working at an advanced level were permitted to prescribe following a long consultation process in 2018 (Blaber et al. 2018).

From the inception of early 'nurse prescribing' as more professionals developed prescribing status, this practice became known as 'non-medical prescribing'. Prescribers who are not medics (doctors and dentists) are now referred to as either independent or supplementary prescribers under the umbrella context of non-medical prescribing. Extended formulary prescribing no longer exists, since being withdrawn by the NMC in 2006 (NMC 2006). Community practitioner nurse prescribers remain in practice and are still undergoing educational programmes to prescribe from the Nurse Prescribers' Formulary with or without a specialist practice qualification such as district nursing.

Barriers to Independent District Nurse Prescribing

Despite the development and growth of independent prescribing by district nurses, there are still some barriers to this in practice. Some of these are discussed here, but this is not an exhaustive list and you may come across different barriers and challenges to prescribing in your own practice. These barriers are mentioned here for you to consider as you develop as a prescriber in order to give you the opportunity to address them before they become an issue for you in your prescribing practice.

A challenge for some district nurse independent prescribers can be accessing ongoing continuing professional development on completion of the education programme in university (Nuttall 2017). While some district nurses have felt that their university programme has equipped them for prescribing in practice (Bowden 2005), others have identified a need for ongoing CPD and have found this difficult to access (Nuttall 2017). CPD for prescribing varies and it is up to you as a district nurse independent prescriber to access what you feel you need in order to remain competent in practice and to maintain the 67 competencies of the *Competency Framework for All Prescribers* (RPS 2016). This may involve seeking your own CPD activities, employer-led activities, support from colleagues, drug companies, pharmacists and other prescribers, as well as consulting journals and research evidence from clinical guidelines. It is essential that you remember as a district nurse that to omit CPD as a prescriber is the potential to compromise patient safety (Nuttall 2017, Scottish Government 2009).

Maintaining confidence and competence can be an issue for district nurses when they commence independent prescribing practice. Maintaining proficiency in the framework for all prescribers (RPS 2016) as you develop your prescribing practice will help ensure you are competent and safe in your prescribing practice. Your competence as a prescriber will be related to the domains of the *Competency Framework* (RPS 2016) and will include pharmacological knowledge, health assessment and diagnostic skills, prescribing as part of a team, prescribing in a public health context and the monitoring of, auditing of and reflection on your prescribing decisions. Being able to articulate and communicate these areas of prescribing practice with your patients will demonstrate your competence for your ongoing and annual Intention to Prescribe declaration with your employer, and will also help to develop your confidence as a prescriber.

Confidence in your ability as a prescriber will influence your prescribing activity, and this will develop as you gain practice, experience and knowledge in prescribing. Your confidence will start to grow upon completion of your prescribing education programme (Nuttall 2017), and this confidence will be enhanced with your professional accountability as a district nurse.

Sometimes the organisational infrastructure may impede your prescribing practice. As an independent prescriber, you need to ensure that you have the necessary infrastructure to support your prescribing as part of your role. This needs to include prescribing as part of your job description, and having support from your employer, with an agreed scope of prescribing practice. You will need to ensure that adequate insurances are in place to protect you and the public. You must also ensure that your prescribing qualification remains annotated with the NMC and that you are able to demonstrate ongoing competency with this as part of your revalidation.

Pressures in district nursing practice, such as a lack of district nurses, under-recruitment into the service, unbounded referral criteria and an ageing workforce (Oldman 2014; Primary Care Workforce Commission 2015) may add to feelings of there not being suitable recognition given to the time and responsibility that prescribing brings to your district nursing role. While prescribing is a practice that aims to enhance patient-centred timely care, it does affect your professional role as a district nurse. You need to ensure that you have the competence, knowledge and skills to prescribe within your scope of prescribing practice, and to maintain your professional accountability. You also need to ensure that you are able to access the time you need to make safe and effective person-centred shared prescribing decisions. It is your role as a district nurse prescriber to advocate with your employer for time to ensure safe and effective prescribing in practice. Often a non-medical prescribing forum and discussions with managers and non-medical prescribing leads can help facilitate this in a healthcare culture where time is a precious and measured commodity. If you do not have adequate time, competence, skill or knowledge to make a safe and effective prescribing decision, then this should be referred on to another prescriber.

Impact and Benefits of Independent District Nurse Prescribing

The RCN (2014) reports that patients have a high level of confidence and satisfaction with independent nurse prescribing, that there are minimal errors at the hands of nurse independent prescribers, that patient care is improved and that there is increased access to medicines, a reduction in waiting times and a delivery of high-quality care.

Independent prescribing has been identified as one of the main interventions that aids the facilitation of patient-centred care in district nursing practice in a holistic approach to care, improving quality of care (Bowden 2005; Downer and Sheppard 2010; Nuttall 2017). This also benefits the service, as independent prescribing has the potential to manage the many demands on the NHS through the better use of resources, including the time spent with patients to provide a person-centred shared prescribing decision (Nuttall 2017).

With a recognition of the increase in long-term conditions and the pressure the NHS is under to meet the needs of those experiencing multiple long-term conditions, the *Five Year Forward View* (NHS England 2014) set out a vision for NHS staff to work with patients as equal partners to provide more control and choice in their care for those experiencing long-term conditions. As this model of care is adopted in practice, district nurses will find themselves working in a more proactive than reactive way in collaborative responses to help manage health and social care needs, whilst meeting service and national agendas such as admission avoidance and self-management. Independent prescribing by district nurses is a key practice that will help meet these agendas, as part of the community workforce providing a variety of care needs to those living at home (Queen's Nursing Institute 2015).

The contemporary aim of district nursing is to employ expert clinical knowledge, clinical assessment, therapeutic relationships and the navigation of complex health and social care systems in a preventative and supportive approach to care (Bliss 2012; Edwards 2014; Kraszesski and Norris 2014), and independent prescribing is a practice that will enhance the facilitation of such aims in holistic and person-centred approaches to care. At the centre of district nursing are the needs of the often older patient who requires attentive, compassionate and responsive care at a time of ill health and dependency, and independent prescribing is a practice that can enhance this.

Independent prescribing has been an important development in district nursing, allowing for new roles, autonomy and smoother service delivery in the provision of holistic patient-centred care. It has also provided value for money in finite healthcare markets (Bowden 2016).

Independent prescribing is evolving in district nursing to meet the needs of the populations and communities it serves. Independent prescribing by district nurses is becoming more common, and the apprenticeship agenda is at the time of press being developed for practice. It is sure to grow, as the NMC annotation of the V300 independent prescribing is identified and recognised as central to this specialist practice district nursing qualification.

Conclusion

This chapter has considered the differing annotations of prescribing and how these have evolved in contemporary healthcare. The history and background to prescribing by district nurses has been discussed, as well as how non-medical prescribing has developed from this. Barriers to prescribing practice for district nurses have been considered, as well as ways these can be addressed in practice. The benefits and impact of independent prescribing by district nurses has been reviewed.

Key Points of This Chapter

- District nursing has a long history in the UK.
- There are a plethora of terms and titles in prescribing practice that, as a prescriber, you need to be aware of for reasons of safety and efficacy.
- Maintaining competence and confidence in your prescribing practice as a district nurse is essential for patient safety, as is ensuring you have the support and infrastructure to support your prescribing practice.

> ◆ Independent prescribing by district nurses has the potential to enhance the patient experience of care, especially for those with long-term conditions, by facilitating safe and effective, timely patient-centred personalised care.
> ◆ Independent prescribing by district nurses offers an opportunity to meet policy agendas for long-term conditions, ensure cost efficacy in finite healthcare markets and ensure smoother service delivery.

References and Further Reading

Blaber, A., Morris, H. and Collen, A. (2018) *Independent Prescribing for Paramedics*. Bridgwater: Class Professional Publishing.

Bliss, J. (2012) Developing a district nursing workforce with advanced skills for care at home. *British Journal of Community Nursing* 18(3): 128–129.

Bowden, A. (2016) The expanding role of nurse prescribers. *Prescriber*. Available at: https://onlinelibrary.wiley.com/doi/abs/10.1002/psb.1469 (last accessed 28 January 2020).

Bowden, L. (2005) The impact of nurse prescribing on the role of the district nurse. *Nurse Prescribing* 3: 79–86.

British National Formulary (BNF) (2019) *BNF 77 March–September 2019*. London: The BMA and The Royal Pharmaceutical Society.

Clegg, A. (2001) Nurse prescribing: Origins and implementation. Available at: www. https:/nursinginpractice/com/article/nurse-prescribing-origins-and-implentation (last accessed 14 August 2019).

Cope, L. C., Abuzour, A. S. and Tully, M. P. (2016) Non-medical prescribing: Where are we now? *Therapeutic Advances in Drug Safety* 7(4): 165–172. Available at: www.https://ncbi.nih.gov.pmc/articles/PMC4959632/ (last accessed 26 February 2020).

Courtenay, M. and Griffiths, M. (2010) *Independent and Supplementary Prescribing: An Essential Guide*. 2nd edn. Cambridge: Cambridge University Press.

Department of Health (DoH) (1989) *Report of the Advisory Group on Nurse Prescribing (Crown Report)*. London: The Stationery Office.

Department of Health (DoH) (1992) *Medicinal Products: Prescription by Nurses and Others Act*. London: The Stationery Office.

Department of Health (DoH) (1999a) *Making a Difference*. London: Department of Health.

Department of Health (DoH) (1999b) *Review of Prescribing, Supply and Administration of Medicines (Crown Report)*. London: The Stationery Office.

Department of Health (DoH) (2001a) *The Health and Social Care Act*. London: The Stationery Office.

Department of Health (DoH) (2001b) *The NHS Plan, a Plan for Investment, a Plan for Reform*. London: Department of Health.

Department of Health (DoH) (2005a) *Nurse and Pharmacist Prescribing Powers Extended*. London: Department of Health.

Department of Health (DoH) (2005b) *Written Ministerial Statement on the Expansion of Nurse Prescribing and Introduction of Pharmacists Independent Prescribing.* London: Department of Health.

Department of Health (DoH) (2006) *Our Health, Our Care, Our Say.* London: Department of Health.

Department of Health (DoH) (2007) *Optometrists to Get Independent Prescribing Rights. Press Release.* London: Department of Health.

Department of Health (DoH) (2013) *The Medicines Act 1968 and the Human Regulations Order.* London: Department of Health.

Department of Health and Social Security (DHSS) (1986) *Neighbourhood Nursing: A Focus for Care (Cumberlege Report).* London: The Stationery Office.

Downer, F. and Sheppard C. M. (2010) District nurses prescribing as nurse independent prescribers. *British Journal of Community Nursing* 15: 348–352.

Edwards, N. (2014) *Community Services. How They Can Transform Care.* London: The King's Fund.

King's Fund (2017) What is social prescribing? Available at: https://www.kingsfund.org.uk/publications/social-prescribing (last accessed 15 August 2019).

Kraszewski, S. and Norris K. (2014) The modern renaissance of district nursing. *Primary Health Care* 24(9): 26–30.

Luker, K. A., Austin, L., Hogg, C. et al. (1997) Nurse prescribing, the views of nurses and other health care professionals. *British Journal of Community Health Nursing* 2: 69–74.

Luker, K. A., Austin, L., Hogg, C. et al. (1998) Nurse-patient relationships: The context of nurse prescribing. *Journal of Advanced Nursing* 28(2): 235–242.

Medicines and Healthcare products Regulatory Agency (MHRA) (2009) *Revised Statement on Medical and Non-medical Prescribing and Mixing of Medicines in Clinical Practice.* London: MHRA.

NHS England (2014) *Five Year Forward View.* London: NHS England.

NHS England (2016a) *Allied Health Professions Medicines Project.* London: NHS England.

NHS England (2016b) *General Practice Forward View.* London: NHS England.

NHS England (2019) Social prescribing. Available at: https://www.england.nhs.uk/personalisedcare/social-prescribing/ (last accessed 15 August 2019).

NHS UK (2017) Who can write a prescription? Available at: www.https://nhs.uk/common-health-questions/medicines/who-can-write-a-prescription (last accessed 14 August 2019).

Nursing and Midwifery Council (NMC) (2006) *Standards for Proficiency for Nurse and Midwife Prescribers.* London: NMC.

Nuttall, D. (2017) Nurse prescribing in primary care: A metasynthesis of the literature. *Primary Health Care Research and Development* 19(1): 7–22.

Oldman, C. (2014) The district nursing service: A national treasure. *British Journal of Community Nursing* 19(8): 394–395.

Primary Care Workforce Commission (2015) *The Future of Primary Care. Creating Teams for Tomorrow.* London: Health Education England.

Queen's Nursing Institute (2015) *Value of District Nursing Specialist Practice Qualification Report*. London: Queen's Nursing Institute.

Royal College of Nursing (RCN) (2014) *RCN Factsheet. Nurse Prescribing in the UK*. Available at: www.https://rcn.org.uk/about-us/policy-briefings/pol-1512 (last accessed 14 August 2019).

Royal Pharmaceutical Society (RPS) (2016) *The Competency Framework for All Prescribers*. London: The Royal Pharmaceutical Society.

Scottish Government (2009) *An Evaluation of Nurse Prescribing in Scotland*. Edinburgh: The Scottish Government.

University of Stirling (2006) History and background to nurse prescribing. Available at: https://ihcs4u.bournemouth.ac.uk/extnurse/Materials/unit1/2_history_background.htm (last accessed 14 August 2019).

Chapter 2

Assessing Health: History-taking and Consultation

Hannah Ingram

In This Chapter

♦ Introduction
♦ Health assessment
♦ Assessment and consultation
♦ Consultation models
♦ Wider determinants of health
♦ Age, sex and constitutional factors
♦ Individual lifestyle factors
♦ Social and community networks
♦ General socio-economic, cultural and environmental conditions
♦ 'Must dos' for safe prescribing
♦ Conclusion
♦ Key points of this chapter
♦ References and further reading

Introduction

This chapter aims to provide a context for health assessment for prescribing practice. This will include concepts of history-taking and consultation styles for prescribing practice. As an experienced district nurse, you will have a wealth of personal experience in your area of practice. The assessment and consultation skills learnt as part of your professional registration are well practised and you are an expert in your field of specialist practice; however, your skills may need to be refined as you take on the role of an independent prescriber.

For most new independent prescribers, across the disciplines, the focus of health assessment, history-taking and consultation skills will be on analysing and reflecting on your current framework of assessment and consultation style, and identifying adaptations you may need to make to support your prescribing decisions. Traditionally, nurses have not adopted a consultation-style approach to assessment of patients and have focused on a holistic assessment of need.

This holistic approach has been to ensure that all physical, emotional, spiritual and social needs of the patient are considered and addressed in district nursing practice. While this is indeed best practice and patient-centred, prescribing brings another context to the health assessment of patients.

Health Assessment

The purpose of any health assessment is to gather a history. The health assessment process is an opportunity for the patient–practitioner relationship to develop and deepen.

However, paradoxical to the holistic assessment of district nursing practice and intrinsic to health assessment in a prescribing context is the need to have an outcome of a diagnosis or differential diagnoses, made through clinical reasoning of the findings of the assessment processes. As you will be aware, the key to making an accurate diagnosis on which to base your prescribing decision is eliciting a good history (Blaber and Harris 2016).

Clinical reasoning is the identification of problems or symptoms that the patient 'presents' with. This will include the identification of any abnormalities in the findings of any examinations undertaken. The skilled practitioner will then link the findings to the underlying pathophysiology in order to establish a set of explanations of causes for such abnormalities. Through this process of hypothetical deductive reasoning (Elstein and Schwartz 2002), the skilled practitioner can create a hypothesis to form a set of differential diagnoses for interpretation. By considering the 'differentials', a working diagnosis can then be formed by reviewing findings with the available evidence base. It is the skilled and experienced clinician who is able to direct a sensitive and nuanced history through relevant questioning in order to elicit an accurate history on which to base their prescribing decisions.

As clinical reasoning and clinical decision making are complex and multi-faceted in district nursing practice, they will be discussed in more depth in **Chapter 3**.

There are a number of factors that support health assessment and clinical reasoning in district nursing practice. These include:

♦ The patient's story
♦ Multi-morbidity
♦ Medication and drug history
♦ Polypharmacy
♦ Altered pathophysiology
♦ The wider determinants of health.

These may be well known to you; however, it is worth revisiting what resources are available to you in formulating a hypothesis and diagnosis in prescribing practice. As already identified, the key to making an accurate diagnosis is through an accurate and thorough assessment and history.

Obviously, the patient's story will inform your clinical reasoning, should they be able or willing to tell you what the problem is − if not, prescribers may have to rely on information from third parties such as family or friends, when available, whilst considering the legal and ethical implications of this. The examinations and investigations you choose to carry out in your assessment processes will be based on your initial findings and will help build up a picture of what is occurring with the pathophysiology. For example, if your patient presents with increased dyspnoea and an audible wheeze, then investigation and examination related to respiratory assessment will give a wider picture of what may be occurring.

Assessment and Consultation

As an experienced district nurse, you will adopt the most appropriate assessment style for the patient in a patient-centred approach to your prescribing practice. You will establish from your initial findings, the situational context and the presentation of the patient whether you need to undertake a complete, episodic, follow-up or emergency assessment.

You will elicit information on any life-threatening issues and manage any presenting risks accordingly in any prescribing encounter, as you would in your professional practice. Having managed risk and ensured patient safety, you will move on to undertaking a focused history and physical examination to identify problems and clinical findings.

History-taking in a prescribing context for district nursing practice includes eliciting and identifying a presenting complaint and any associated symptoms and issues the patient may be experiencing. You will also ascertain a comprehensive past medical history and drug history. This will then lead to a physical assessment and review of body systems, as appropriate. In ascertaining presenting complaints and associated symptoms, it may be useful to employ mnemonics as a framework to guide your enquiry, such as SOCRATES to assess pain (AACE 2013).

Further information on the use of mnemonics can be found in **Chapter 3**.

For prescribing practice, it is essential that you can draw on the assessment skills that you have and incorporate a prescribing perspective in doing so to adopt a consultation approach. By doing this, you will be able to facilitate a patient-centred and shared decision-making approach to your prescribing practice. Each consultation for prescribing will take an individual stance or approach depending on the patient, the context and the presenting complaint (see **Case Study 2.1** and **Case Study 2.2**). Each consultation should follow the same principles:

♦ Patient-centred
♦ Professional
♦ Evidence-informed
♦ Shared decision making.

The two case studies below highlight the importance of the care being delivered by the practitioner who makes the initial diagnosis. This avoids undue distress and frustration caused by multiple practitioners carrying out the same assessment to enable them to prescribe. These case studies demonstrate the effectiveness of prescribing, enabling the district nurse to make patient encounters truly patient-centred, professional and evidence-based. In both cases, the shared decision making was between the district nurse and the patient.

Case Study 2.1

You are a district nurse independent prescriber and are visiting Mabel. Mabel has bone metastases from advanced breast cancer and also experiences high cholesterol and has a chronic leg ulcer. She lives alone in a very remote rural area and has limited social contact with her estranged son. Mabel's daughter visits monthly to bring shopping and is reluctant to provide any further help. She has refused carers.

Mabel is being treated with methotrexate and currently reports that she takes half an aspirin (150 milligrams) once a day, as her Great Aunt Dot swore by this for a long and healthy life, which she gets over the counter via her daughter.

Mabel is experiencing pain from her leg ulcer and has requested a prescription of a non-steroidal anti-inflammatory drug (NSAID) such as ibuprofen, as she reports she does not like paracetamol.

You are able to identify as a district nurse independent prescriber that methotrexate and ibuprofen are high-risk medications.

NSAIDs and aspirin increase the absorption of methotrexate. Methotrexate causes folic acid depletion and this may need to be supplemented.

Plan:

Advise Mabel to stop the aspirin immediately and provide information as to why.

Discuss the evidence with Mabel and agree to refer to the GP/cancer services for review following this information.

Undertake a pain score. Discuss with Mabel why she does not like paracetamol. Does she have accurate information about this medication, can she take it properly, does she realise the increased benefit of regular administration, is the formulation she has right for her, does she need a different formulation (e.g. dissolvable preparations)?

Case Study 2.2

Bob is 90 years old and has atrial fibrillation, hypertension, diabetes and a leg ulcer. He takes warfarin (he is unsure of the dose), ramipril 5 milligrams once daily, metformin 1 gram TDS and ibuprofen 200 milligrams TDS. Bob refuses to take a statin. He is allergic to penicillin.

On assessment, you identify an infection to the leg ulcer which is hot, exudating and painful. He has a pyrexia of 38°C. Bob also reports some loose stools.

There is a caution with the prescribing of antibiotics with warfarin. Warfarin is a high-risk drug. When prescribing antibiotics, always refer to local guidelines and the BNF for safe use concomitant with warfarin and for antimicrobials safe for use in the case of a penicillin allergy.

Plan:

Undertake a wound assessment and reach the decision that systemic antibiotic therapy is required. Seek advice from BNF/pharmacist/local formulary on the safe and appropriate antibiotic to prescribe, liaise with GP and ascertain eGFR before prescribing antibiotics (eGFR = 60 ml/min/1.73 m^2).

Prescribe clarithromycin 500 milligram tablets BD for 7 days (clindamycin contra-indicated in diarrhoeal states).

Deprescribe ibuprofen as this should not be used in conjunction with warfarin due to increased risk of bleeding. Ascertain a pain score and prescribe paracetamol 1 gram, six hourly, for 14 days if Bob is unable to obtain this over the counter. Report to GP and document. Ensure Bob has the relevant information regarding this and is able to identify the risk.

Loose stools may be the unwanted effect of metformin; check what formulation Bob is using as a modified release may improve symptoms. Undertake an abdominal and GI assessment to rule out other differential diagnosis.

(BNF 2019; PHE 2017)

Consultation Models

There are a plethora of consultation models available to use for prescribing practice that can assist the practitioner in undertaking a structured consultation, drawing on their communication skills and experience whilst developing prescribing practice. Not all available models of consultation can be discussed here; however, a few are outlined to provide a basis for consulting with patients, with recommendations for prescribing practice.

 There is further discussion on consultation models and approaches in **Chapter 3**.

The general purpose of a consultation model in the context of independent prescribing for district nurses is to give you a structured approach to take a nuanced and focused history on which to base your differential diagnosis, which will inform your prescribing decision. These can be particularly useful for district nurses as they commence independent prescribing practice. Traditionally, as district nurses, we have undertaken assessment processes where the patient takes the lead in 'telling their story'. While this is best practice in district nursing, in prescribing it is important to elicit all the facts of the presenting complaint and related issues in order to make a safe and effective prescribing decision. This may mean that you need to lead the assessment in a consultation approach in order to elicit the information you need.

The Pendleton et al. (1984) model offers a patient-centred approach to a prescribing consultation in discussing their ideas, concerns and expectations (ICE). This includes:

♦ Defining the reason for attending
♦ Considering other problems
♦ Choosing an appropriate plan with the patient
♦ Achieving a shared understanding with the patient
♦ Involving the patient with managing the plan
♦ Using time and resources effectively
♦ Establishing and maintaining a relationship.

Neighbour (1987) outlines similar contexts in his model, building on that of Pendleton et al. (1984), where he acknowledges that intentions and plans of the prescribing consultation may not always turn out as expected. He also incorporates some reflective practice to prescribing in his model:

♦ Connecting (relationship building)
♦ Summarising (reaching a shared understanding, considering ICE)

- Handing over (shared decision making in the prescribing plan)
- Safety netting (what to do if things don't go to plan)
- Housekeeping (reflective practice).

A commonly used and well-known model of consultation is the Calgary-Cambridge model (Silverman et al. 1998):

- Initiating the session
- Gathering information
- Building a relationship
- Explanation and planning
- Closing the session.

This model includes shared decision making and a patient-centred focus through the patient setting the agenda without relinquishing all of the decision making by the prescriber. It offers structure and direction; however, it does not consider reflection as part of prescribing practice, or the wider governance and strategic perspectives of prescribing practice.

The National Prescribing Centre (NPC 1999) formulated a framework to guide the seven principles of safe prescribing practice to assist in decision making (see **Figure 2.1**), which has been used by nurse independent prescribers as a consultation and step-by-step approach to prescribing practice since they have been able to undertake prescribing in practice.

Consideration of the Patient

- Who is the patient?
- Is it appropriate for you to prescribe for them within your scope of prescribing practice?
- What is the presenting complaint?
- How long has it been going on?
- Has anything been tried already?
- Is the patient taking any other medication that may affect your decision?

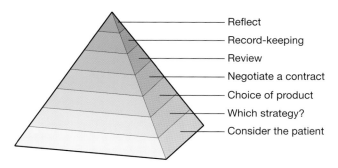

Reflect
Record-keeping
Review
Negotiate a contract
Choice of product
Which strategy?
Consider the patient

Figure 2.1 – The prescribing pyramid
Source: NPC (1999).

Which Strategy?

♦ Consider if there is a working diagnosis that has been established.
♦ Is a referral onto another healthcare professional/prescriber indicated?
♦ Is a prescription needed?
♦ Is patient expectation a factor?
♦ What treatment options are available?

It is important to remember that a prescription should only be issued if there is a genuine need. It should only be issued if, on balance, this is the best option for the patient at the time of presentation and within the context of this presentation.

Considering the Product

The National Prescribing Centre (NPC) (1999) offers the mnemonic EASE to assist in deciding how to select a product to prescribe:

♦ E: How **effective** is the product?
♦ A: Is it **appropriate** for this person?
♦ S: How **safe** is it?
♦ E: Is the prescription cost-**effective**?

Negotiate a Contract

♦ Has shared decision making taken place?
♦ Does the patient know how to take this medication correctly and safely?
♦ What safety netting has taken place; do they know what to do and who to contact if something goes wrong?

Review the Patient

♦ Consider what follow-up is needed.
♦ Consider repeat prescribing, and your prescribing role and scope of prescribing practice.

Record-keeping

♦ Consider the NMC and your employer's requirements for safe and effective contemporaneous record-keeping.
♦ Consider that there needs to be a clear audit trial to inform further prescribing decision making.

Reflection

♦ Reflective practice improves prescribing practice.
♦ Consider what has gone well and what has not gone so well.

♦ Formulate an action plan for your future prescribing practice.
♦ What learning and development needs have been identified?
♦ What can others learn from this?
♦ Who do you need to support you?

The *Competency Framework for All Prescribers* (RPS 2016) (Table 2.1) offers a structured, patient-centred consultation framework specifically for prescribing practitioners to use, incorporating consideration of prescribing governance issues. It is a consultation model.

The model (RPS 2016) also incorporates the competencies required for all prescribers to achieve safe and effective patient-centred prescribing. It is these competencies you will need to demonstrate you have achieved when undertaking the independent prescribing course. The NMC expects all prescribing registrants to be able to meet this competency framework (NMC 2018). Therefore, due to the specific prescribing nature of this consultation framework and its mapping to the competencies required for all prescribers, it is highly recommended that this is the consultation framework that is adopted by district nurses undertaking prescribing practice.

The consultation model detailed in Table 2.1 can be used in conjunction with the prescribing pyramid's seven principles (Figure 2.1) to safe prescribing (NPC 1999) as your prescribing experience develops, as this will encourage reflective prescribing practice.

It is important in prescribing practice to refer to your practice experience in making prescribing decisions. As a district nurse, you will have gained a

Turn to **Chapter 12** for more detail on reflective practice.

Table 2.1 – The *Competency Framework for All Prescribers* model

Consultation	Prescribing Governance
1. Assess patient	7. Prescribe safely
2. Consider options	8. Prescribe professionally
3. Come to a shared decision	9. Improve prescribing practice
4. Prescribe	10. Prescribe as a part of a team
5. Provide information	
6. Monitor and review	

Source: Based on RPS (2016).

wide level of experience and knowledge in your area of expertise and this will form the basis of your clinical reasoning and decision making. You will pick up cues from your patients about what they are experiencing through the language that is used, both verbally and non-verbally, and you will be able to interpret this by drawing on your experience and intuition. There has long been a debate about the use of intuition in nursing practice. What I mean to refer to here is 'how you know things' in practice. This can be about cue recognition, from what you may have seen or heard in your experience; it can also relate to the assimilation of theoretical knowledge from the classroom into practice situations. The key here is not to use 'intuition' or whatever way of describing 'what you know you know' in prescribing practice in isolation, but to utilise your experience concurrently with your experience, the clinical presentation and assessment findings and the evidence base available to you.

Turn to **Chapter 3** where clinical decision making is explained further.

Wider Determinants of Health

A key element of health assessment on which to base safe and effective prescribing decisions is the consideration of the holistic needs of patients and the influences on the health of the individual. As prescribers, we need to consider the wider determinants of health. Dahlgren and Whitehead (1991) formulated the concept of the wider determinants of health when looking at strategies to promote social equity in health. The model has utility today in considering influences on health and how this may affect your prescribing decision making in practice; see **Figure 2.2**.

Think about:

It is useful to think about how these wider determinants of health may influence your prescribing decisions in your prescribing practice as a district nurse.

Looking at **Figure 2.2**, consider how each determinant may have an influence on your decision making as an independent prescriber.

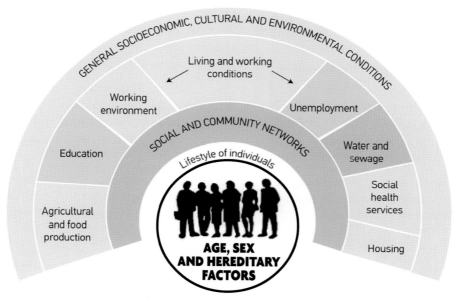

Figure 2.2 – Wider determinants of health

Source: Dahlgren G, Whitehead M (1991). *Policies and Strategies to Promote Social Equity in Health*. Stockholm, Sweden: Institute for Futures Studies.

Age, Sex and Constitutional Factors

Considering age, sex and constitutional factors at the centre of **Figure 2.2**, we can identify that these factors have an impact on our health. For example, as we age, we become less well and more prone to disease, and our sex will pre-dispose us to certain health and disease risk factors. When considering prescribing decisions, you will need to consider a patient's age and sex.

Ageing and Multi-morbidity

As people age, they are more likely to develop co-morbidities complicating the course of intervention and treatment that can be offered; this will be a major consideration in your prescribing decision making. The presence of two or more long-term conditions is now considered multi-morbidity; this is associated with a poorer quality of life and a greater use of health resources, such as medicines and appointments.

Prescribing decisions in multi-morbidity need to be patient-centred. Special attention should be paid to patient choice and quality of life outcomes. When considering prescribing in multiple pathologies, it is advisable to consider the evidence available for single disease pathology and discuss this with the patient. Evidence sources such as NICE treatment guidelines are a valuable resource, but it must be remembered in prescribing practice that these evidence sources are compiled from research into people experiencing single disease pathology. It is essential to remember that the patient with multiple long-term disease pathology is likely to be an expert in their health, and their opinion should be sought and included in any decision.

In prescribing for symptom relief in multi-pathology, it is essential to consider any treatment for its effectiveness and its evidence base for use. This needs to include the stopping and reducing of medicines and monitoring the effects. Non-pharmacological interventions for symptom relief should also be considered in multi-pathology to reduce the treatment burden.

When considering prescribing for predicted risk of future disease, there is special consideration of multi-pathology as it is not always advisable to increase the medication and treatment burden on those with multiple chronic health needs (BNF 2017).

Turn to **Chapter 7** for more information on evidence-based practice.

Polypharmacy

Polypharmacy is the prescribing of multiple items to one person (Duerden et al. 2013). This usually refers to items of medication, but in the UK and especially for district nursing practice this can refer to dressings, appliances and blood monitoring equipment, as well as supplements. Initiating one medication for one complaint will have a potentially huge impact on another condition. Concurrent with multiple co-morbidities in age, people will inadvertently have multiple medications to treat and manage these conditions, which will result in polypharmacy.

Again, the more medications people take, the more problems they are likely to experience due to their ability to manage multiple medicines effectively; they may be more likely to experience interactions and adverse effects from polypharmacy. In addition, as people age, they will be more likely to have had a previous experience of an adverse drug reaction, reducing the choice of treatments you have to consider when you prescribe.

While the term polypharmacy implies criticism of the number of items prescribed for one person, it is essential in multi-morbidity and for older people that a plethora of drugs and associated appliances is used to treat the conditions experienced. Therefore, it is important to consider the need for appropriate polypharmacy and problematic polypharmacy (Duerden et al. 2013) when prescribing for older people and for multi-morbidity as a district nurse independent prescriber.

Appropriate polypharmacy is the prescribing for a patient with complex or multiple conditions where the medication has been prescribed in accordance with best evidence and has been optimised in its use. The intention of the combination of medicines is to promote and maintain quality of life and optimum symptom control, and to minimise harm (Duerden et al. 2013).

Problematic polypharmacy is when there is an inappropriate amount of multiple medications prescribed or when the intended benefit of the prescribed drug has not been achieved. Polypharmacy can be problematic when treatments are not evidence-based, when the risk of harm outweighs the benefits, when there is a risk of drug interactions, when the amount of medicines is unacceptable to the patient, when the regime is too complicated for the patient to follow or when medicines are prescribed to treat the side effects of other medicines (Duerden et al. 2013).

Deprescribing

Deprescribing is when a prescriber reduces or discontinues medications or changes their doses in order to manage polypharmacy (BNF 2017). Due to the issues outlined above, de-prescribing should be part of your routine clinical prescribing assessment strategy, as **Case Study 2.3** highlights. Any de-prescribing decisions should be undertaken in partnership with patients in a shared decision-making approach. This facilitates a person-centred approach to prescribing practice, but also encourages the taking of medicines to their best effects with the least likelihood of an unwanted outcome.

Case Study 2.3 highlights the importance of taking a thorough history and reviewing all medications prescribed, whether they be long-standing prescriptions or additional medications for short-term use. Patients will sometimes only mention medications that they take regularly over a long period of time.

Altered Pathology in Ageing

Age also brings with it altered pathology and end organ failure. Of particular concern in prescribing practice is liver and renal disease due to pharmacokinetics.

Liver Disease

Liver disease can alter the response of drugs and, as such, prescribing in all patients with liver disease should be kept to a minimum. Problems particularly occur in patients experiencing jaundice, encephalopathy and ascites. Metabolism by the liver is a route of elimination for many drugs; however, liver disease has to be quite severe to alter the metabolism of drugs. Routine liver function tests are not a reliable source of estimating the liver's capacity to metabolise drugs and therefore should not be routinely undertaken. Similarly, it is not possible to ascertain to what extent an individual may metabolise a drug. Therefore, prescribing for liver disease should be undertaken with extreme caution and by prescribing practitioners working in the speciality of hepatic care (BNF 2019).

Case Study 2.3

You are visiting Sheila, a 78-year-old woman who has recently had a total knee replacement. You have been asked to visit to remove the clips to the wound and undertake an assessment. During your assessment, you ascertain that Sheila was diagnosed with hypertension following her pre-operative assessment and was commenced on Ramipril 6 weeks ago by her GP. Sheila complains of an increasingly persistent dry irritant cough. She also discloses she thinks she may be constipated as she has not had her bowels open for 3 days and has increasingly painful abdominal cramps.

Sheila has no known allergies. She is taking 2.5 milligrams daily of Ramipril, co-dydramol 20/1000 milligrams every 4–6 hours.

Sheila reports a pain score of 2–3/10.

Sheila lives with her daughter.

Sheila reports no chest pain, no chest tightness, no cyanosis, no oedema, no pursing of lips and no sore throat, and is able to continue activities of daily living. She reports that her cough is dry and irritating and has been persistent for the last month.

On respiratory assessment, there are bilateral vesicular chest sounds.

Sheila's observations are satisfactory:

    HR 96
    BP 125/65
    Blood glucose 4.8
    RR 18
    Temp 36.8°C
    SpO2 98%

Differential diagnosis:

Query cough secondary to commencement of ACE inhibitor (Ramipril).

Constipation secondary to co-dydramol.

Plan:

De-prescribe co-dydramol and consider prescribing paracetamol 1 gram QDS if Sheila is unable to buy these over the counter. Give advice on not using co-dydramol and paracetamol preparations simultaneously.

Refer to GP for review of ACE inhibitor and prescription of an ACE2 if this is outside of your scope of prescribing practice.

Contact patient's GP and document findings.

Other important points to note in liver disease when making prescribing decisions and reviewing medications include the following:

♦ Reduced clotting increases the sensitivity to oral coagulants such as warfarin from a prolonged prothrombin time, caused by reduced hepatic synthesis of blood clotting.
♦ Reduced protein binding in hypoproteinaemia in severe liver disease can cause toxicity of highly protein-bound drugs such as phenytoin.
♦ Oedema and ascites can be exacerbated by drugs that cause fluid retention such as NSAIDs and corticosteroids.
♦ In severe liver disease, some drugs can impair brain function and cause hepatic encephalopathy. Sedatives, opioids and diuretics should be avoided, as should any drug that causes a risk of constipation (BNF 2019).

Renal Disease

Prescribing in renal disease should also be undertaken with caution. However, even if suspected due to the clinical picture, renal function should always be checked before prescribing any medication that may require drug modification in renal disease.

The main issues encountered in renal disease and impaired renal function can cause problems for many reasons. These include the following:

♦ Reduced excretion by the kidneys may cause toxicity of the drug.
♦ Sensitivity to some drugs can be increased in renal disease, even if there is no impairment to an individual's elimination of the drug.
♦ Some drugs can be ineffective when there is a reduction in renal function.
♦ People who experience renal disease and poor renal function may not be able to tolerate the side effects of some medications (BNF 2019).

Many of these problems can be minimised through effective prescribing of reduced doses or the replacement of drugs with different medicines. Patient-centred prescribing is of value; listening to the patient and their experiences of the issues encountered and the side effects of their medications will lead to safe and effective prescribing practice in renal disease. Patients who experience renal disease and therefore require special consideration in prescribing practice are likely to require follow-up and review.

Turn to **Chapter 5**, where prescribing in special groups is discussed in more depth.

Individual Lifestyle Factors

Each individual's choice of lifestyle and associated lifestyle factors will have an impact on the prescribing decisions you make. Lifestyle behaviours not only have an impact on health and health outcomes, but also on the medications and options you have to prescribe.

You will have considered a social or family history as part of your assessment strategy; however, for prescribing in district nursing practice, you will also need to take a wider perspective on lifestyle factors, as this is a critical aspect on which to make your prescribing decisions. All illness treatment and interventions should be seen in the context of the individual and should include consideration of beliefs, personality and spirituality. Occupation, environment, interests and behaviours, such as smoking and alcohol consumption, have a profound impact on health and disease.

Similar to eliciting a presenting complaint as part of your assessment strategy, there are mnemonics for social assessment and history-taking that need to be considered for safe and effective holistic person-centred decision making in prescribing practice. These can be seen in **Box 2.1**.

Smoking

Smoking is a lifestyle choice with now well-known risks to poor health outcomes as it is one of the most common causes of lung disease and the main cause of chronic obstructive pulmonary disease (COPD). As such, smoking may often be hidden from prescribing practitioners by patients, carers and families due to the stigma that has become associated with it. Assessing smoking-related activity is part of any assessment. For example, evidence of smoking, or smoking in the home will help inform your clinical diagnosis and affect the decision to

---

Box 2.1 – Mnemonics for social assessment

SAFE	S: Smoking A: Alcohol F: Food E: Exercise
HELP	H: Housing E: Employment L: Living/dependants P: Pets
HAT	H: Hobbies A: Activities T: Travel

Source: Nutall and Rutt-Howland (2011).

---

prescribe oxygen due to the associated risk of fire. Similarly, smoking needs to be considered in patients with long-term conditions. Not only does smoking increase the severity of dyspnoea and disease progression in pathologies such as heart failure and COPD, it is also an associated cardiovascular risk in type 2 diabetes (Meerabeau and Wright 2011) and can worsen the symptoms of multiple sclerosis (Wingerchuk 2012). Such issues may affect your prescribing decision making in terms of what medication and titration you may have to consider for individual patients when prescribing for smokers in these pathologies. Likewise, it is essential to consider if the drug you wish to prescribe is affected by smoking. For example, clozapine used for psychosis in Parkinson's disease may need dose adjustment should smoking be started or stopped during treatment (BNF 2017).

Alcohol

Alcohol misuse is a huge public health issue in the UK. Alcohol misuse in the elderly population is increasing (Holley-Moore and Beach 2016) and, as such, has risk factors for prescribing practice. Again, alcohol consumption may be hidden from prescribing practitioners due to the social stigma it carries, and if it is reported in a holistic assessment, it may be difficult to ascertain an accurate picture of consumption and frequency. Alcohol intake needs to be considered in prescribing practice as it has many risk factors when taken concomitant with certain medications and can cause hepatotoxicity; caution and consideration are required in the prescribing decision-making process.

Due to its anticoagulant affect, alcohol needs to be considered when prescribing drugs with the same properties, such as aspirin and warfarin, as excessive anticoagulation can occur, resulting in a risk of bleeding. Likewise, alcohol use has a gastric risk and the prescribing of gastric irritants such as NSAIDs should be done with caution, even with a proton pump inhibitor.

Alcohol use in the elderly can increase the risk of falls; therefore, prescribing drugs that can exacerbate the risk of falling, such as diuretics and anti-hypertensives, should be given special consideration and regular monitoring of the patient should occur. Undertaking a falls risk assessment is a useful resource to guide decision making in prescribing when falls are a consideration.

Alcohol also has sedative properties and therefore can exacerbate the effects of narcotics and tranquilisers, and this intensification should be avoided. Alcohol can also cause dehydration, and this can affect the therapeutic use of some medicines, as well as affecting the metabolism and elimination. Risk of dehydration should be considered in your assessment when making prescribing decisions where alcohol misuse is suspected. Alcohol can have interactions with common medications that you may wish to prescribe. For example, when prescribing antibiotics, it is essential to consider alcohol use, as not only can the consumption of alcohol reduce the therapeutic effect of some antibiotics, but it can also result in serious and life-threatening interactions with antibiotics such as metronidazole.

This is by no means an exhaustive list of issues to consider in terms of smoking and alcohol in prescribing practice as a district nurse. However, it does highlight the need to be aware of the effects and impacts that these lifestyle risk factors may have on the medications that make up the scope of your prescribing practice.

Food

Dietary requirements have an influence on prescribing practice. Food may be a prescribed item itself for those with special dietary requirements, or as a nutritional supplementation, and this can be an issue when considering the cost to the patient of prescriptions. The increase in the use and need of foodbanks for patients needs to be considered in prescribing practice and when making social prescriptions of nutritional intake. Patients may not wish to use certain medications if they contain animal products such as gelatine or have been used in animal testing, and you may need to reconsider your decision making in a patient-centred approach.

Similarly, some drugs that you may wish to prescribe within your scope of practice may have interactions with some food sources and patient counselling will be required to ensure that the concomitant use will be avoided. Consumption of grapefruit or grapefruit juice must be avoided with some medications, such as statins, calcium channel blockers and cytotoxic drugs, as it can increase the therapeutic level of the drug, leading to toxicity and increased side effects.

Antacids are widely used in the population for heartburn and are often not reported as drugs in a medication review, as they can be purchased over the counter. It is important to assess lifestyle factors such as diet and food intake to elicit such problems as heartburn, acid reflux and indigestion. Long-term use of antacids can cause a mild magnesium deficiency which can go undiagnosed. Magnesium is required for the absorption and usage of calcium in the bones and can be a cause factor in the increase in osteoporosis in people who use these medicines for a long time. Consideration should be given to patients who present in your prescribing practice the long-term use of antacids and proton pump inhibitors, especially women.

Exercise

Exercise is a healthy lifestyle choice and should be encouraged in a public health perspective to prescribing practice, where appropriate for your patient group in district nursing practice. It should be considered that exercise can have some implications for your prescribing practice. Statins can cause reversible myositis and therefore this severe muscle pain will impact on the ability to exercise. Statin use will need to be considered in patients presenting with pain requesting analgesia for muscle pain.

Lactic acidosis is the build-up of lactic acid in the muscle tissue that results from intense exercise. Some medications cause lactic acidosis, such as metformin in type 2 diabetes and some HIV drugs. Metformin should not be given to diabetics with hepatic or renal disease as this increases the risk of lactic acidosis. This may have considerations for your prescribing practice if you are presented with a patient with diabetes or HIV exercising for positive health outcomes and complaining of intense muscle pain.

Housing

Housing may impact on your prescribing decisions in terms of people's ability to access medication and in the storing of medication. Elderly, frail people with mobility issues may not be able to regularly access medication and may have to rely on others for this. This should be considered when considering your prescribing decision in terms of the amount of a medicine you wish to prescribe. Issues may occur if there is a lack of suitable storage facilities in the home, such as refrigeration for insulin or vitamin B12. Likewise, if there is a risk of misuse of medicines due to other residents in the home and the storage of high street value drugs such as codeine, narcotics or tranquilisers, this will need to be factored into your prescribing decision.

Some presenting complaints such as recurrent chest infections may have a root cause of housing issues rather than respiratory disease and as such are worth exploring. Poor ventilation, damp, pet hair and lack of heating are all factors to consider in making your prescribing decisions, especially if this occurs remotely from the patient's home.

Employment

Although district nurses have traditionally cared for older housebound populations, changing demographics and in-service provision have resulted in the need to consider employment in this population group.

Employment will have an impact on any social or medical prescribing you may undertake in practice. A patient's employment (or lack of) will influence their ability or willingness to engage with treatment regimens that you may wish to consider. People aiming to take medications whilst working need to consider their ability to do so prior to commencing medications. This decision making in partnership with patients will increase adherence to medication regimes and prevent waste. The working environment may not be conducive to the timing of tightly controlled regimens, such as QDS insulin whilst maintaining set teaching schedules. The environment may not lend itself well to clean or aseptic techniques, such as injectables or intravenous therapy for antibiotics required on a building site. Similarly, a lack of employment or a low income may prevent some people from wishing to engage in treatment regimes that have a cost involved. This may not be restricted to prescription costs or costs of equipment such as dressings, but may include some foodstuffs or supplements that are required to complement the prescribed drug regime. Some people without employment may be experiencing poverty and may not wish to have health practitioners in their home environment.

In terms of employment, it is also paramount to consider the wider issues of the prescribed regime you wish to consider. This includes whether the prescribed medication will affect the patient's ability to work when this is of financial or psychological importance to them. This could include the sedative effects of a medication such as benzodiazepines and some antidepressants such as sertraline on their ability to drive or concentrate. There are legal penalties for driving or being in control of a vehicle when under the influence of controlled or prescribed drugs, so caution must be taken by the prescriber and the patient (BNF 2019). The government provides information on its public websites on the rules and regulations regarding this. This could also include the side effects experienced being so severe that it makes fulfilling the job role challenging. For example, severe rhinitis experienced as a side effect of citalopram for a dentist would make their job difficult, as would requiring regular toilet breaks for a community worker or air cabin crew experiencing diarrhoea from antibiotic therapy.

Again, employment will have an impact if there are other prescribed regimes for the patient's condition that require attendance at appointments concurrent with any prescribed medication regime. This needs to be considered when making shared patient-centred prescribing decisions. For example, treating chronic or a new onset of musculoskeletal pain with analgesia may be complemented by a course of physiotherapy that the patient may find difficult to attend due to their employment pattern. This also needs to be considered in the management of depression where antidepressant medication is an adjunct to talking therapies or prescribed exercise regimes that are now seen to be the more effective course of action for the illness (Meerabeau and Wright 2011; NICE 2009).

Paradoxically, it also needs to be considered when making prescribing decisions if the patient you are treating is legitimising their 'sick role' in a quest for medication (Meerabeau and Wright 2011) and to avoid employment or work. This will be elicited by the skilled practitioner as part of the health assessment process, but it is paramount to work in partnership with the patient and reach a shared prescribing decision. That is not to say that any prescriber should feel pressured into making a prescribing decision at a patient's request; if in doubt, seek support from your wider team such as pharmacists and medical GP prescribers.

Living/Dependants

Living can incorporate lifestyle factors, as previously discussed. This concept can also include daily routines for people experiencing and managing long-term conditions or coping with the effects of ill health. For example, a person may not wish to leave their home or socialise if they feel embarrassed or stigmatised by their long-term condition, which may impact on any prescribing intervention you make. Some people with chronic leg ulceration experience malodourous exudate and may not wish to attend clinic appointments or adhere to the prescribed treatment or exercise therapy due to this. Psoriasis may result in skin-shedding in public, causing embarrassment to the sufferer, resulting in social isolation; treatment regimes can also be part of the problem as well as the solution and must be discussed in shared decision making with the patient (Meerabeau and Wright 2011). Some older people living at home with ill health may not want visitors to the house as they are embarrassed by the medical equipment in the home and this can lead to social isolation.

Someone living with COPD or heart failure may have a specific daily routine that helps them to cope with and alleviate dyspnoea. This needs to be considered when deciding on new treatment regimes and interventions, as the person with a long-term condition is the expert in managing their health, has done so for a long time and has often maintained a pattern of living that enables their independence or optimal level of independence in coping with disease pathology (Snodden 2009).

Considering dependants not only concerns those who have children to care for whilst requiring medication regimes, but also people who undertake care as unpaid work. This may involve looking after older people or even animals. It is important to maintain a person-centred approach to prescribing, as care of others will often take precedence over care of oneself for people who undertake caring roles (Phillips 2007). This can impact on prescribing decisions as people may find it impossible or too much of a challenge to undertake a medication regime that interferes with their existing responsibilities, such as their employment, as already discussed. To make a patient-centred and shared decision, the areas such as unpaid care work and daily living routines need to be incorporated into the prescribing decision.

Pets

Pets are an important consideration in the social assessment process. They are often a highly valued part of people's lives and therefore must be considered in making prescribing decisions. This is not just as part of the caring role or people seeing pets as dependants. Pets can be a contributing factor to the exacerbation of disease in illness such as asthma. Allergies to animal fur can initiate or exacerbate eczema and rhinitis. While to a practitioner, it may seem sensible to avoid such triggers, to a patient, the pet may be the one element of their lives that brings them joy and quality of life. Therefore, it is important to consider how the inclusion of pets can be facilitated in daily living whilst considering medication and social prescribing that allows the patient to live well. For example, this may include the prescription of increased inhaler therapy in asthma and social prescribing of encouraging the patient to keep the cat out of the bedroom. Alternatively, it could be the prescription of some topical steroid therapy for eczema, with regular emollient therapy and encouraging the patient to cover their arms in light cotton fabric whilst petting their furry friend.

Hobbies and Activities

Much of what has been discussed above can also be attributed to the consideration of an individual's hobbies and activities when considering prescribing decisions. The key ethos in social assessment is considering the person as an individual, with their own life and routine, and with a role in making a shared decision about a prescribing intervention that is going to be conducive to them maintaining their chosen or set lifestyle and routine. Of course, that is not to say that as a prescriber, you should not take the opportunity to provide education or health promotion where it is indicated in your prescribing consultation regarding health and lifestyle behaviours. Making Every Contact Count is a health policy strategy that utilises everyday interactions to encourage and help people make healthier choices and achieve positive long-term outcomes through behaviour change (NHS England 2014), and this should be incorporated into prescribing consultations and practice by all prescribers.

It is also of value to consider any sporting activity that your patient may undertake as a hobby, as certain medicines that you may consider prescribing may have unwanted effects on their performance or may negatively impact on any doping testing that may be undertaken. This needs to be considered for those patients undergoing cancer treatments who may be trying to maintain health and fitness through sport. Care is needed as well as a shared decision-making approach. Professional athletes and sports personnel will usually be well informed about any medications that they can or cannot take. Any prescriber who colludes in the provision of drugs or treatment to enhance sporting activity may have their professional registration questioned; however, this does not preclude the intention to improve or protect health (BNF 2019).

Travel

Travel remains an important issue for prescribing practice for district nurses. More and more frequently, older people are able to travel with family to visit loved ones in other countries despite living with long-term and complex health problems. Additionally, people receiving treatment for cancer may be within the district nurse caseload where prescribing and travel are concomitantly considered. Travel will influence prescribing decisions in terms of whether it will be possible to incorporate a prescribing decision into travel plans. Travel history and foreign travel must also be considered as part of a full health and social assessment. Recent travel may provide an indicator as to the cause of symptoms and presenting health complaints.

The BNF offers a guide to travel vaccinations. These guidelines change frequently and therefore the most current and up-to-date information should be sought when counselling a patient with this advice or eliciting a health history. Health information on overseas travel for professionals can be accessed at www.nathnac.org.

People travelling to the UK from abroad may have medications that do not have a MHRA licence for use here, and therefore cannot be prescribed should they need further supplies. There may be similar medications available here, but excipients may be different, so care and caution are required in prescribing practice. Prescribing as part of a team is imperative in these instances and collaboration with pharmacists and medical and specialist colleagues is required. It may be indicated that a medication review and new regime has been commenced. In the absence of information on excipients in the most up-to-date BNF or in the product literature, contact the manufacturer, as it is essential to ensure that the details are correct (BNF 2019). Information on product literature can be accessed at www.medicines.org.uk/emc.

Social and Community Networks

Dahlgren and Whitehead's (1991) model considers social and community networks. This is significant in prescribing practice as these factors will influence a person's ability to participate in their prescribed treatment plan. For example, older people may require a support network in order to be able to participate in shared decision making and undertaking a prescribed medication regime. This support network could be either informal, in the form of family support for decision making, or more formal, in the form of third-sector initiatives such as community transport to access follow-up appointments or medication. This could also include formal networks such as the community pharmacy and medication delivery systems. This is not limited to the elderly; people undergoing therapy for rehabilitation for intravenous drug use often rely on formal community pharmacy initiatives for medication management to support success. Insulin-dependent diabetics and people at the end of their life often need formal community networks such as district nursing services as well as informal family and carer support. Investigating these social and community networks will assist you in person-centred decision making as it will elicit what options a person may have on which to base an informed choice in relation to their care.

General Socio-economic, Cultural and Environmental Conditions

Work, unemployment, food, housing and living conditions have been discussed as part of the social assessment in prescribing practice. Wider strategic considerations identified by Dahlgren and Whitehead (1991) include the following.

Education

Health literacy has a big impact on prescribing practice. A person's knowledge about their condition and the treatment required will assist in the shared prescribing decision-making process. Good health literacy will also impact on a patient's willingness, motivation or ability to undertake a medication regime as prescribed, or whether there could be some deviance from the prescribed regime due to a lack of understanding.

Younger people may not see their health as a priority and may not seek help in the first instance, especially for potentially embarrassing problems such as pilonidal sinus. People in education may have reasons for not seeking health professionals on a regular basis if they are transient between addresses and may let problems lapse. As younger people in education may change addresses from term to holiday time, this can make the follow-up of prescribing decisions harder to facilitate.

Once referred to and under the care of a district nursing team, younger people may be harder to follow up to review care and prescribing decisions due to a lack of understanding and importance placed on health. For example, younger people receiving IV therapy for cellulitis or an abscess may not appreciate the risks of sepsis. It is the responsibility of a skilled practitioner to elicit the presenting complaint in a patient-centred consultation in order to identify the problem and plan a collaborative treatment regime.

Water and Sanitation

This is an important consideration in all areas of healthcare practice, as well as in prescribing practice. Consideration of access to clean sanitised areas and clean water supplies is important in prescribing decisions. It is essential to consider if the person has access to adequate facilities with which to self-care effectively, but also to undertake prescribed medication regimes. For example, a patient with psoriasis requiring regular wet bandages and emollient application will need washing facilities in order to be able to undertake this. Sanitation is an important consideration in primary care when making prescribing decisions. It needs to be considered if the person is able to maintain independence in living with an addition medication or treatment regime and if it is safe to do so. The risk to visiting health and social care professionals in unsanitary living accommodation needs to be considered, as well as the risk to the person. With more and more intravenous therapy being delivered in the home, such as IV antibiotics for cellulitis, it is essential that the risk/benefit ratio is calculated as part of a risk assessment where there is potential harm that could come to the patient if the home were not suitable for visiting healthcare professionals to deliver aseptic care.

Healthcare Services

A lack of access to healthcare services may put pressure on some prescribers when a number of complaints are saved for one short consultation, as with increased demand on health services, the patient may have trouble in accessing appointments. This may also result in patients asking for prescribed medication that is outside the scope of your prescribing practice. The district nurse prescriber needs to be confident in refusing to prescribe when this occurs in order to ensure patient safety and to protect their registration.

Similarly, it is essential to consider in your prescribing decision making what health and social care services are available to your patient group, and where

Box 2.2 – 'Must dos' for safe prescribing

- Is this the right patient? Check your records are the person's records! This sounds simple, but mistakes are easy to make and hard to resolve.
- Is the patient's history and presenting complaint appropriate for your scope of prescribing practice? If not, refer on.
- Check the patient's weight where appropriate for safe prescribing.
- Ascertain allergies or interactions.
- Ensure that the patient is not experiencing a condition that may be exacerbated by the medication you wish to prescribe (e.g. NSAIDs with peptic ulcer, antacids, grapefruit and interactions).
- Ensure that the patient does not need a modified or reduced dose (e.g. if a child, elderly or in renal failure).
- Inform the patient of nuisance and serious side effects, and what to do and who to see in the event of these occurring.
- Pregnancy is a high-risk group to prescribe for. Always check for pregnancy in women of childbearing age.
- Be sure you have knowledge of the clinical evidence-based guidelines and local formularies.
- Consider de-prescribing and the high-risk danger drugs which have an increased chance of interactions (such as warfarin, NSAIDs, phenytoin, bisphosphonates and antacids).

you can refer them to for adjuncts to the medication you prescribe. Each local area will commission different services and this can be a challenge for practitioners to keep a handle on. Offering patients advice on wider holistic and social interventions that they may be able to access, whether commissioned or not in the local area, will ensure that the public health initiative of making every contact count is undertaken within your prescribing role (NHS England 2014), rather than just the provision of a prescription. **Box 2.2** includes some key points or 'must dos' to guide you in every patient encounter you have in a prescribing context.

Conclusion

In health assessment and consultation for prescribing practice, a key theme that has been discussed in this chapter is the process of a patient-centred and shared decision-making approach to your prescribing practice. While undertaking prescribing practice as a district nurse, there is a high chance that there will be pressure put upon you to undertake prescribing decisions quickly from all stakeholders with whom you will come into contact. As an independent prescriber, it is imperative that you maintain your scope of prescribing practice, prescribing only medicines and drugs that you are competent and confident to prescribe, and for disease processes and pathophysiology that you are familiar with. Prescribing and de-prescribing is a complex business that requires time, caution, attention and practice. Using a consultation framework that is evidence-based, such as the *Competency Framework for All Prescribers* (RPS 2016), will ensure a structured and cohesive approach to your prescribing practice, where you will be able to demonstrate your ability to meet the competencies in a safe and effective way.

Key Points of This Chapter

♦ Shared decision making and a patient-centred approach are central to obtaining a thorough, accurate health assessment of your patient.
♦ Various models and frameworks have been explained that may assist you.
♦ It is not always essential to prescribe; it is just as important to consider other options.
♦ Always use and review the 'must dos' for prescribing.

References and Further Reading

Association of Ambulance Chief Executives (AACE) (2013) *UK Ambulance Services Clinical Practice Guidelines 2013 Pocket Book: Pain Assessment Model.* Bridgwater: Class Professional Publishing.

Blaber, A. Y. and Harris, G. (2016) *Assessment Skills for Paramedics.* 2nd edn. Maidenhead: Open University Press.

British National Formulary (BNF) (2017) *The British National Formulary 74, September 2017–March 2018.* London: BMJ Group.

British National Formulary (BNF) (2019) *The British National Formulary 77, March–September 2019.* London: BMJ Group.

Dahlgren, G. and Whitehead, M. (1991) *Policies and Strategies to Promote Social Equity in Health.* Stockholm: Institute of Future Studies.

Duerden, M., Avery, T. and Payne, R. (2013) Polypharmacy and medicines optimisation, making it safe and sound. London: The King's Fund. Available at: https://www.kingsfund.org.uk/sites/default/files/field/field_publication_file/polypharmacy-and-medicines-optimisation-kingsfund-nov13.pdf (last accessed 26 February 2020).

Elstein, A. S. and Schwartz, A. (2002) Clinical problem solving and diagnostic decision making: Selective review of the cognitive literature. *British Medical Journal* 324(7339): 729–732.

Holley-Moore G. and Beach, B. (2016) *Drink Wise, Age Well: Alcohol Use and the Over 50s in the UK.* London: International Longevity Centre.

Meerabeau, L. and Wright, K. (eds) (2011) *Long-Term Conditions, Nursing Care and Management.* Chichester: Blackwell Publishing.

National Institute for Health and Clinical Excellence (NICE) (2009) *Depression in Adults (Update). Depression: The Treatment and Management of Depression in Adults. National Clinical Practice Guideline 90.* London: NICE.

National Prescribing Centre (NPC) (1999) *Nurse Prescribing Bulletin. Signposts for Prescribing Nurses: General Principles of Good Prescribing.* London: NPC.

Neighbour, R. (1987) *The Inner Consultation: How to Develop an Effective and Intuitive Consulting Style.* Lancaster: MTP Press.

NHS England (2014) *An Implementation Guide and Toolkit for Making Every Contact Count: Using Every Opportunity to Achieve Health and Well Being in the NHS.* London: NHS England.

Nursing and Midwifery Council (NMC) (2018) *Realising Professionalism: Standards for Education and Training. Part 3: Standards for Prescribing Programmes.* London: NMC.

Nutall, O. and Rutt-Howland, J. (2011) *The Textbook of Non-medical Prescribing.* Oxford: Wiley-Blackwell.

Pendleton, D., Scofield, T. and Tate, P. (1984) *The Consultation: An Approach to Learning and Teaching.* Oxford: Oxford University Press.

Phillips, J. (2007) *Care.* Cambridge: Polity.

Public Health England (PHE) (2017) *Management of Infection Guidance for Primary Care Adapted for Local Use. Brighton and Hove CCG, High Weald Lewes and Havens CCG.* London: Public Health England/NHS England.

Royal Pharmaceutical Society (RPS) (2016) A *Competency Framework for All Prescribers.* London: RPS.

Silverman, J., Kurtz, S. and Draper, J. (1998) *Skills for Communicating with Patients.* Oxford: Radcliffe Medical Press.

Snodden, J. (2009) *Case Management of Long-Term Conditions: Principles and Practice for Nurses.* Chichester: Blackwell Publishing.

Wingerchuk, D. M. (2012) Smoking: Effects on multiple sclerosis susceptibility and disease progression. *Therapeutic Advances in Neurological Disorders* 5(1): 13–22.

Chapter 3

Decision Making for Prescribing

Amanda Blaber, Hannah Ingram and Jennifer Gorman

In This Chapter

- ◆ Introduction
- ◆ An overview of decision making in the community
- ◆ Problem solving and critical thinking
- ◆ Decision making models and theory
- ◆ Human factors in decision making
- ◆ Influences on prescribing
- ◆ Practical application for District Nurses
- ◆ Principles of good prescribing
- ◆ Use of IT systems in prescribing decisions
- ◆ Conclusion
- ◆ Key points of this chapter
- ◆ References and further reading.

Introduction

This chapter will examine the role of problem solving and critical thinking as a means to make evidence-based effective decisions. Theoretical aspects of decision making will be briefly examined and considered in the light of relevant human factors theory.

Practical application of the theory will be explored using case studies, examining the principles of good prescribing practice and the use of various mnemonics. Finally, the chapter will explore the specific issues of practising as a district nurse and the information technology that is available to assist with prescribing decisions.

An Overview of Decision Making in the Community

As a district nurse, you will often be working alone. This means that you are autonomous in your practice and decision making. However, it is essential to remember when making prescribing decisions in the community, just as with your professional practice, that you are never working in isolation. It is incredibly important to remember that there is a plethora of information and resources available to support your decision making and to aid you in safe and effective prescribing practice.

Mobile devices will give you access to the internet and credible sources of information such as NICE guidelines and the BNF. You will be aware of your local organisational formularies as an independent prescriber and these are often accessible via intranet sources. You will be able to contact a local community or hospital pharmacist for advice and support as well as the patient's GP. Family and carers of the patient can often provide a rich source of information to aid your decision making, as will the patient themselves.

If you are unable to access the information you need to make a prescribing decision, then you should delay the decision making and the prescription until you are able to access the information required that will inform a safe and effective evidence-based decision.

Lone working in the community gives rise to the need to be able to provide a clear account of your decision-making processes so that you can justify prescribing decisions made, and discuss and reflect upon them to improve your prescribing practice. When prescribing as a district nurse you will need to communicate your decision making with an integrated team, such as the GP and other professionals involved. This is not only to update others on prescribing interventions made, but also to further inform subsequent decisions regarding the patient's care by other practitioners and prescribers. Therefore, you must be able to account for the process used in your decision making, and how and why you reached the decision. This will include analysis of all factors you consider in reaching a prescribing decision and the evidence base utilised behind the decision made.

Problem Solving and Critical Thinking

Decision making is one of the most important leadership activities and is at the heart of healthcare management (Marquis and Huston 2017). Before any effective decision can be made, the processes of problem solving and critical thinking should be consciously undertaken. Problem solving is an integral part of the decision-making process. In fact, decision making is the final step in the problem-solving process. This has the potential to be quite a lengthy 'higher-order' thinking process – TIME is the one thing most healthcare professionals lack. It is, therefore, important to note that a decision can be made without the full analysis required in problem solving. The key is to hone your approach and problem-solving formula or theory to make the best possible decision for your patients, within your scope of practice, working environment, knowledge base and the resources available.

Critical thinking and reflection are inextricably linked. In order to evaluate a situation, critical thinking skills should be routinely employed by experienced healthcare practitioners. This will involve a broader scope of analysis than that of problem solving or decision making. This means more complexity for the individual and higher-order reasoning, honest evaluation and both cognitive (knowledge and understanding) and affective (mood, feelings or attitudes) components.

Turn to **Chapter 12** for more on reflective practice.

Theorists (Facione 2006; Marquis and Huston 2017; Pritchard 2006) have cited what they believe to be key characteristics of critical thinkers (see **Box 3.1**). The characteristics may be innate to individuals and come easily when required in a practice situation. It is often wrongly assumed that if an individual does not recognise the traits in themselves, then they will struggle to think critically. This is inaccurate, but a danger of listing characteristics is to damage clinicians' confidence and make them feel inferior to their peers. It is important to note that many of the characteristics listed in **Box 3.1** can be learnt and practised and may not prohibit a clinician from making effective decisions, provided that a proven structured approach is taken.

One of the most dangerous approaches to decision making is the taking of 'shortcuts'. Clinicians – indeed any human being – rely on 'discrete, often unconscious processes' called heuristics (Marquis and Huston 2017). Heuristics

Box 3.1 – Characteristics of a critical thinker

- Open to new ideas
- Intuitive
- Energetic
- Analytical
- Assertive
- Communicator
- Flexible
- Empathetic
- 'Outside the box' thinker

- Caring
- Observant
- Risk-taker
- Resourceful
- Creative
- Insightful
- Willing to take action
- Willing to change
- Knowledgeable.

involves an individual recognising patterns and then being able to solve a problem or reach a conclusion more rapidly. In a healthcare context, a nurse may recognise a presentation of a patient as being familiar to them (as they have seen it previously in other patients) and apply several shortcuts (not fully assessing the patient or assuming certain facts without checking thoroughly) in order to reach a decision about treatment and management more quickly. This approach can be unconscious, so nurses need to examine their practice and self-regulate their tendency to take shortcuts. In short, nurses need to BEWARE HEURISTICS. These 'shortcuts' may work most of the time, but they can sometimes be detrimental to patient care and outcome; see Case Study 3.1.

Case Study 3.1

In this case study, we consider two scenarios where a heuristic prescribing decision is made.

Scenario 1

As a district nurse prescriber, Sarah is visiting Betty in her rest home as the staff have called and reported a change in micturition pattern. Betty is well known to Sarah as she receives regular care and nursing interventions for her diabetes. Sarah is aware that Betty has had repeated urinary tract infections in the past. Sarah assesses Betty and ascertains she does have a lower UTI. Sarah has a clear knowledge of Betty's other medications and the local formulary guidelines and BNF, so makes a quick heuristic decision to prescribe nitrofurantoin 50 milligrams QDS for 3 days.

What Sarah has not considered in making a shortcut decision is Betty's eGFR, which is 40 ml/min, and therefore nitrofurantoin should only be used with caution (BNF 2019). This is because the efficacy of the drug depends on renal secretion of the drug into the urinary tract. In renal impairment, the efficacy is therefore actually reduced.

Scenario 2

Betty is complaining of pain from her venous leg ulcer. She has been feeling under the weather for a few days, complaining of a cold and fever. Pushed for time, Sarah quickly assesses Betty and rules out a wound infection. As Betty has no access to the shops for a few days until her daughter visits again, Sarah decides to prescribe some paracetamol for Betty to help with the pain to her leg ulcer, and arranges delivery with a local pharmacy.

Had Sarah undertaken a full and holistic assessment with Betty before making a heuristic decision, then she would have established that Betty was already taking an over-the-counter cold remedy that contains paracetamol, thus leaving her at risk of an unintentional overdose.

Luckily for Sarah, in her heuristic prescribing decision making she omitted to ascertain Betty's preference for the formulation of paracetamol and had prescribed tablets. When they were delivered, Betty decided not to take them as she was unable to swallow them and required a soluble formulation.

This shortcut time-pressured prescribing practice was not only unsafe, putting Betty at risk, but it was also ineffective as it resulted in a prescribing decision that was not person-centred.

As a means to prevent poor problem solving and as a consequence poor decisions being made, a traditional problem-solving model may be useful (Ignatavicius 2001):

1. Identify the problem
2. Gather data to analyse the causes and consequences of the problem
3. Explore alternative solutions
4. Evaluate the alternatives
5. Select the appropriate solution
6. Implement the solution
7. Evaluate the results

The above seven steps are subject to interpretation and there are many adaptations/versions of problem-solving models for the professional to peruse and critique. A selection of decision-making models is briefly considered in the next section.

Decision-Making Models and Theory

Perspectives of Modern Decision-Making Theory

It is commonly accepted that decision making, in the wider context, relies on the schools of psychology and economics (Johansen and O'Brien 2015). In many industries, 'good enough' decisions are taken, as the costs incurred by exploring and analysing every decision to be made would be prohibitive (Simon 1959). The process of minimising risks and problems is now commonplace. Maximising profits (economics) is less common to the decision-making process in public services such as healthcare. Simon (1959) proposed that people do not always act rationally; they rely on their judgement. The following series of models details the modern development of theories associated with decision making.

Cognitive Continuum (Hammond et al. 1975).

As mentioned above, 'judgement' is central to decision making. The 'quality' of the decision made will depend on the accuracy of an individual's judgement. It will also depend on the individual's ability to 'pick up on' and interpret the 'cues' from any given situation. Hammond (2000) explains that any judgement is a mix of 'task properties' and 'cognitive processes'. Task properties can be

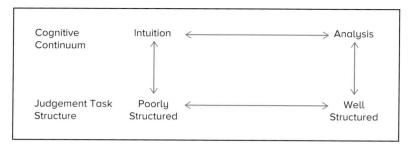

Figure 3.1 – Visual representation of cognitive and judgement task structure continuums

defined as the weighing and combining of information by the decision-maker in order to make judgements. Cognitive processes include both intuition and analysis. Hammond et al. (1975) describe individual preference as not being purely analytical or intuitive, but as usually lying on a cognitive continuum, as shown in **Figure 3.1**.

Hammond et al. (1975) proposed that where a decision-making approach to tasks was poorly structured, it was usually the result of an overly intuitive (less analytical) approach. Where a well-structured approach to decision making was taken, this was usually the result of a more analytical (than intuitive) approach to the decision taken. Our decisions are not usually wholly intuitive or analytical, so the continuum proposed by Hammond et al. (1975) is logical. If individuals are more aware of the dangers of being purely intuitive or analytical, then the decisions made should be more robust. Of course, in healthcare things are often more complex and the type of task will often determine the clinician's type of thinking (intuitive or analytical). The length and type of the clinician's prior experience is another highly relevant variable, as explored by Hamm (1988). Subsequently, the complexity of decision making in nursing was recognised and led to various models of decision making being specifically developed with these complexities in mind.

Analytic Models of Decision Making
The analytic decision-making model assumes that the person/people involved in making any decision is/are thinking rationally and logically. Anyone examining the clinician's decision (after the event) should therefore be able to follow the clinician's logical and rational thinking and come to a similar conclusion/decision. Key parts of this model are the nurse's experience, and their ability to identify situations and to use guiding principles/a set of rules in order to make a decision (Banning 2008). This model does not seem to account for high-stress environments or emotional situations.

Information-processing Approach to Decision-Making
This is based on a hypothetical-deductive analytical method to assist nurses to make decisions. There are four proposed steps (Tanner et al. 1987):
1. Cue recognition/acquisition
2. Hypothesis generation

3. Cue interpretation
4. Hypothesis evaluation

In many cases, nurses have developed and used decision trees/pathways to assess possible outcomes. The accompanying research iterates that decision trees/pathways usually enable nurses to make better decisions; however, it is noted that this model also relies on the nurse possessing a competent, well-developed knowledge base (Banning 2008; Manias 2004).

Intuitive-humanist Model of Decision Making

The main principle of this model asserts that there is a major difference between the 'novice' nurse and the 'expert' nurse in terms of their ability and way they make decisions. The model proposes that the expert nurse does not rely on analytical principles (seeing a situation as a series of parts) in order to understand a situation or to take action. An experienced nurse sees and uses 'patterns' or recognises similarities between situations they have experienced in the past. It is recognised that in nursing many situations are complex, uncertain and have not been encountered previously, therefore intuition is an important part of decision making, but should be used with caution by more 'novice' nurses. The more experience a person has, the more situations they have to draw upon in order to create several options, prior to making their final decision. King and Clark (2002) agree that as nurses gain experience, the quality of their analysis around their decision making improves. The dangers of over-relying on patterns was addressed at the beginning of this chapter.

Multidimensional Clinical Decision-Making Model

As the title suggests, this model takes into account that the clinical decision making of nurses is multidimensional and complex in nature (O'Neill et al. 2005). It takes account of the previous models and the novice-expert clinical reasoning model (O'Neill and Dluhy 1997). The main features are:

♦ Investigating patient-specific prior data
♦ Risk assessment and reduction
♦ Nursing standards of care
♦ Situational elements affecting decision making
♦ Salient concerns
♦ Triggers for hypothesis selection
♦ Subsequent nursing action.

The main basis for this model is a computerised decision-making support system, where pattern recognition and information processing are key themes. The fact that this model has its origins in computer programs highlights the complexity of decision making in the clinical environment.

An important choice for nurses is to find a model that is evidence-based yet easily understandable and, more importantly, useful in the clinical environment. The IDEALS model (Facione 2006) may be a reasonable compromise and act as a 'self-check'.

IDEALS Model

The main parts of the IDEALS model are presented below, with associated questions which can be adapted for your place/type of work:

- Identify the problem – 'What is the real issue here?'
- Define the context – 'What are the facts, what is known, what are the circumstances?'
- Enumerate the choices – 'What are the most realistic three or four options?'
- Analyse the options – 'All things considered, what is our best course of action?'
- List the reasons explicitly (to yourself or to your team) – 'Let's be clear, why are we making this choice?'
- Self-correct – 'Okay, before we/I take action, let's look at this again. Did we/I miss anything? What did we/I miss?'

It is also important to recognise individual variation in decision making. Some of these points may seem logical and obvious, but it is important to ensure we are all aware of our own potential causes of bias and shortcomings, and the effect these may have on the decisions we make. All of our decisions are based on our own value system, which may consciously or unconsciously influence our decision making. Once the information is gathered, the generation of alternatives is encouraged. It must be remembered that our own values may also influence our perceptions and therefore may affect the information-gathering process. Gathering information may be an individual or team approach; a more detailed gathering of data may be achieved through a team approach. Once information is gathered, many of the models encourage generation of options/choices before committing to a final decision. Our own value system may inhibit the creation of options/choices; therefore, team decisions (even small teams) may generate a wider, more diverse range of choices (Facione 2006). The next part of the chapter will explore some of the human factors that may affect decision making.

Human Factors in Decision Making

'Human factors' is a relatively 'young' subject area within healthcare, yet it is an established discipline within 'safety critical' industries such as aviation. Human factors, also known as 'non-technical skills', has been recognised by the National Health Service (NHS) as a discipline to be researched, adopted and adapted in order to provide optimal human performance and decision making in healthcare. This will also afford the reduction of risk to patients (National Quality Board 2013).

Communication is at the heart of healthcare and of every encounter with patients, families and colleagues. Issues with communication are one of the main causes of complaints to the NHS (Ford 2015), so regardless of the experience of the nurse, communication needs to be consistently evaluated and reflected upon. Hence, a reminder of communication styles has been included in this chapter.

Communication Styles

Depending on the texts read, there are several styles of communication. This chapter will briefly address the four types, omitting the manipulative style, which is not appropriate for healthcare environments or situations. Individuals may have a natural tendency towards one style, but different styles of communication can be practised and refined.

Passive/Submissive Communication
As reflected by the title, individuals who possess this style of communication do not like conflict. Therefore, they seek to please others by being apologetic in their communication, speaking softly and avoiding eye contact. Passive/submissive communicators fail to assert themselves and may feel anxious, sometimes low in mood and resentful as their needs are not being met. It is common for passive communicators to avoiding expressing themselves – their opinions or feelings.

Aggressive Communication
Such communicators will often stand up for themselves or express their thoughts by becoming angry or physically aggressive if they do not get their own way. Their approach is to disregard all other views, considering them not worth considering or as incorrect. They may have fixed eye contact, a raised volume of speech and an intimidating posture. Their style may be to humiliate and use control over others, forcing people to agree with them. This is unprofessional in front of patients and will be detrimental to building a rapport with anyone.

Assertive Communication
This is a clear, respectful and appropriate communication of feelings and thoughts. People using this style are able to advocate for their rights without showing aggression. Key features of people who are assertive in their communication style are high self-esteem and the ability to listen to others (without interruption), to appear in control of themselves and to maintain good eye contact. This is thought to be the most effective communication style. It facilitates us being able to take care of ourselves and show respect for others, and ensures good relationships (Matthews 2018).

Situational Awareness

The concept of 'bandwidth' is becoming more widely appreciated as an important idea for healthcare staff to be aware of. A nurse will only be able to hold and assimilate a certain volume of information at any one given time; this concept may be termed the nurse's 'bandwidth'. A nurse's working memory can only process a limited about of new information (Riem et al. 2012). This is a separate entity to long-term memory.

Once a nurse's bandwidth capacity has been reached, they will start to lose situational awareness and suffer tunnel vision. The following are symptoms of full bandwidth capacity in a highly stressful, acute environment:

♦ Becoming task-focused
♦ Losing sight of the 'bigger picture'
♦ Increased stress levels
♦ Increased panic
♦ Not hearing anything that is said
♦ Losing peripheral vision.

These symptoms/feelings will result in a lack of productivity or efficiency for the individual and team. Bandwidth can be expanded by education, experience and continued exposure to your clinical environment. This is a concept that is crucial to consider when orientating new staff to any new discipline or clinical area.

Teamworking

In 2017, the Royal College of Nursing (2017) stated that the ability and 'health' of a team have a direct correlation with patient safety. Teamworking is often superseded by leadership in terms of importance. Teamworking is essential for high-quality care, is invaluable and is a crucial human factor and one sometimes taken for granted.

When working in teams, people will demonstrate different strengths and weaknesses, take on different roles within the team and be required to be flexible and responsive to the dynamic and changing environment in which they are working. Teamworking can present many challenges and there is not always a place for many 'leaders'; the concept of 'followship' is worth mentioning.

'Followship' is an art in itself, as with leadership. It requires people to be adept at following direction, allowing a leader to lead, while remaining proactive, engaged in their role and supportive. It is best practice for a leader to share information with the team in order to receive feedback and respect others' knowledge, thoughts and opinions.

Clinical leadership is a commonly addressed subject on both pre- and post-registration nursing courses. The wide range of identified leadership styles is outside the remit of this chapter. Leadership is identified as one of the non-technical skills that constitute human factors, and should be respected and honed by nurses as they gain their registration and as their careers progress.

Escalating Concerns

Unfortunately, things do not always run smoothly with our working environments or our interactions with patients and families. If you have a genuine concern and think an individual's practice requires challenging, then the mnemonic PACE may be useful (Besco 1999):

♦ **P**robe
♦ **A**lert
♦ **C**hallenge
♦ **E**scalate.

This is a four-phase method of escalating concerns using an assertive communication style. The aim is to highlight concern to the individual being challenged. Using PACE should enable a structured, professional and assertive approach, which should ensure that a difficult and potentially unsafe/dangerous situation can be avoided. **Case Study 3.2** highlights how PACE may be used in a district nursing situation.

Case Study 3.2

Sally is observing her colleague, Anne, assessing and prescribing medication for a patient, Mrs Patel. You listen to the patient assessment and hear Mrs Patel declare that she is allergic to penicillin. Anne is talking to Mrs Patel and is about to prescribe amoxicillin.

Did you hear Mrs Patel say she is allergic to penicillin?

Sally is 'probing' to see if Anne is aware of the 'bigger picture', as well as highlighting her concerns in a simple, non-confrontational manner. Anne seems distracted and ignores Sally. Sally steps up her assertiveness, with a slight increase in volume:

Can we ask Mrs Patel to repeat what she said to you earlier about allergies?

Anne may be displaying signs of cognitive overload for whatever reason, and may be focused on writing the prescription and moving on to the next patient. Anne appears very stressed and is not listening to Sally. Although Sally has raised concerns, she now needs to 'challenge' Anne in a louder, assertive tone:

Please stop writing that prescription, as Mrs Patel is allergic to the medication you are about to prescribe.

This 'challenge' is not acted upon and Anne is fixated on the prescription. Sally may need to raise her assertive level even more, highlighting the issue further. It is best to use tactile stimulation, such as a hand placed lightly on the shoulder and addressing Anne by name, in an assertive but professional manner:

Anne, STOP writing that prescription for Mrs Patel, she cannot take amoxicillin as she is allergic to penicillin.

Anne will take note of this, hopefully realising her loss of situational awareness and admitting to herself and Mrs Patel that she is overwhelmed and had misplaced her focus. Due to Sally's style of communication and escalation, no harm was done, professionalism was maintained, and Anne was supported and not embarrassed in front of Mrs Patel.

Influences on Prescribing

It is important to be mindful of influences on your prescribing decision making, and reflecting on these will inform your development and proficiency as a district nurse prescriber and will aid safe and effective prescribing practice.

Think about:

What influences do you think there are on your prescribing practice as a district nurse?

Some influences on your prescribing practice will be more obvious than others. There are several influences on prescribing decision making, some of which are considered here. This is not an exhaustive list, as every patient, situation and context of prescribing is unique and will have differing influencing factors:

- The patient
- Family and carers
- Your experience and knowledge as a district nurse and a prescriber
- The expectations of other people
- The pharmacy industry
- Local formularies
- Organisation's policy and procedure
- NICE guidelines
- Colleagues
- Attitudes and opinions.

The patient and their wishes will influence your prescribing decision making, not only through the presenting complaint and the individual concomitant factors, but also with their own perspective, health beliefs, health literacy and ideas, concerns and expectations. Reaching a shared decision with your patient is essential in prescribing practice, as this will optimise the engagement with the treatment and optimise the medicines use.

Family and carers will often influence your decision making. They often hold a solid knowledge base of the patient and will be able to supply you with specific information that will influence your prescribing decision. For example, they will be able to report on issues such as swallowing, dexterity and beliefs held that can assist you in making a person-centred decision. Family and carers may also have strong ideas and expectations about what you should be doing and prescribing for their loved one. It is essential to remember that although you may want to meet the expectations of others, you must work within your scope of prescribing practice and only prescribe within this. You must also consider your role as a district nurse and as an independent prescriber, and act within your professional code (NMC 2019) and within the limits of your practice. In difficult situations, remember you can access the wider integrated team and seek support and advice if you are unsure of a safe and effective resolution for the patient.

Your experience and knowledge as a district nurse will influence your prescribing decisions. Working autonomously in the community setting caring for people in their own homes will have given you a wide experience of how people manage and adapt to their medication regimes. This will influence your practice as an independent prescriber. For example, you will have an awareness of prescribing practices and cautions for those living alone, for those with limited mobility and for those with limited resources. These are important social and economic factors to consider when making prescribing decisions around medications that can cause falls or alter a person's cognitive state, when access to a bathroom is needed rapidly or frequently or when the prescribing decision may result in an inability to maintain work patterns or will incur a large cost to the patient.

The patients you assess as a district nurse prescriber may have an expectation of receiving a prescription from you. This can be a challenge to manage in some instances where the patient is adamant that they require a prescription. Again, it is important to ensure that a shared decision is reached; this may involve you taking the time to explain and advise your patient of your decision making and providing them with the evidence base behind it to enhance their understanding. If having undertaken an assessment you have made an evidence-based decision not to prescribe, you should not change your mind based on patient expectations and any pressure exerted on you. **Case Study 3.3** highlights some of the potential challenges you may face as an independent prescriber.

Alternatively, patients may expect you to prescribe a particular treatment but your own prescribing decision based on the available evidence does not support this. It may be that the patient desires this treatment due to a lack of knowledge or understanding of the pathology of their condition. Again, taking the time to explain your rationale and to signpost the patient to resources on how you have reached this decision can help them understand the person-centred approach to your decision making.

The pharmaceutical industry may have an influence on your prescribing practice. Although the industry has an important role in medicine by providing new and innovative products and drugs, a transparent relationship must be maintained

Case Study 3.3

You are visiting Vera at home in her warden-assisted accommodation. She complains that the chronic pain she has to her venous leg ulcers is not controlled with paracetamol. She asks you to prescribe her some dihydrocodeine. On further consultation and assessment, you discover that Vera is asking for this medication as Mavis two doors down has recently been prescribed this medication post-operatively and swears it has relieved all her pain, so she would like the same please.

Taking the time to explore this with Vera, you can advise her on the contraindications of dihydrocodeine such as for those with a history of constipation – a common, painful and frequent complaint of Vera's. You are also able to establish that Vera is not taking her paracetamol as prescribed and you can advise her on the improved therapeutic effect of taking this medication regularly.

with prescribers. This ensures that prescribing decisions are not influenced by promotional information or products and that they remain evidence-based and person-centred. This will ensure patient trust and that safe and effective prescribing decisions are made (BMA 2019).

There is controversy over how pharmaceutical companies' marketing targets prescribers and how this is likely to influence patient care. Pharmaceutical companies often offer free lunches and gifts from representatives who call at your base (BMA 2019). Some representatives can be particularly persistent in trying to gain access to you to promote their merchandise, especially if they are aware of your prescribing status. To avoid undue influence by the pharmaceutical industry, you should avoid accepting representative lunches and gifts and avoid meeting them unless this is part of a wider decision and context made by your employing organisation (BMA 2019). Your employing organisation may have a policy on dealing with the pharmaceutical industry, with which you should comply.

Further NHS best practice guidelines on dealing with the pharmaceutical industry can be found at: https://www.networks.nhs.uk/nhs-networks/joint-working-nhs-pharmaceutical/documents/dh_082569.pdf.

Turn to **Chapter 7** for more on assessing clinical trial data for yourself.

Local formularies and national guidelines such as NICE provide a valuable evidence-based resource that will influence your decision making in prescribing practice. However, it is important to note that a limitation of NICE guidelines is that they only consider single disease pathologies and not multi-morbidity. In district nurse prescribing practice, you are likely to be dealing with and prescribing for patients with multiple comorbidities, and therefore you need to be aware of how prescribing for one disease pathology will have implications for another pathology. You need to be certain of your knowledge, evidence base and decision making in this context, and seek support when the decision is out of your scope of prescribing and professional practice.

Your organisational local formularies provide an evidence-based and cost-effective resource for your prescribing practice. Some organisations will allow you to prescribe outside the formulary they have provided if you are able to provide an evidence-based rationale for doing so; others will not allow you to prescribe outside of the local formulary. Therefore, you should be fully aware of your organisational policy and procedures around this issue and ensure that you act accordingly within the terms of your employment and NMC registration.

Colleagues' attitudes and opinions can have an influence on your prescribing practice. As part of your prescribing practice, you may attend forums with more experienced district nurse prescribers where prescribing scenarios, problems, successes and challenges are discussed. Reflecting on the experiences of others can help inform your learning and practice as a novice prescriber, and your prescribing experiences will inform the learning and practice of others too. However, it is important to remember that not every prescribing situation is the same and you need to make patient-centred evidence-based decisions based on your own assessment findings for the individual patient, rather than simulate or repeat a prescribing decision made by someone else in a similar context.

As part of a wider district nursing or integrated care team, as a prescriber you may experience situations where members of the team ask you to prescribe for a patient they have seen based on their assessment findings. This is not good practice and you should be very wary of doing this as you have not made the assessment on which to base a prescribing decision (see **Chapter 9** for more information). The General Medical Council (GMC 2013) offers clear guidance on best practice and how to avoid pitfalls in prescribing at the request of other clinicians.

You need to prescribe professionally and safely, and ensure that you accept personal responsibility for prescribing and understand the legal and ethical implications of doing so (RPS 2016). Only ever prescribe within the limits of your practice and within your scope of prescribing practice and do not feel under pressure to prescribe at the request of another practitioner. Remember that you are not prescribing in isolation – there are other resources and support systems available to you, and to other team members, to ensure safe and effective decision making for patient care.

Practical Application for District Nurses

As a district nurse, it can sometimes be useful to employ strategies that support your decision making in prescribing practice. You will already be undertaking assessments of your patients based on a nursing model or framework adopted by your employer and service. However, using strategies and frameworks that support decision making in practice will help demonstrate an evidence-based and structured approach to your prescribing practice that will ensure safe and effective patient-centred prescribing.

There are a number of strategies that you can adopt to demonstrate a structured approach to your decision making. Some are considered here, although this is not an exhaustive list.

Mnemonics

A practical way of ensuring robust decision making can be through the use of mnemonics. These can be a useful way for prescribers to ensure the key considerations are made for each clinical encounter. There are a wide variety of mnemonics available and these cover more than just the actual act of prescribing, taking on the history-taking and physical assessment findings too (see Box 3.2).

It is important to remember that although these can be useful to aid your decision-making processes in a prescribing context, they should not be used as an aside to a full and holistic patient-centred assessment. There are wider considerations that will influence your prescribing decision making, such as environmental, social and economic factors. See **Chapter 2** for more information.

The Competency Framework for All Prescribers

An excellent resource for demonstrating a safe and effective structured decision-making process is the *Competency Framework for All Prescribers* (RPS 2016).

The *Competency Framework for All Prescribers* gives a structured format on which to base your prescribing decision making. A competency is a quality or characteristic that reflects effective performance and can be described as a melange of skills and knowledge. Competencies help individuals and organisations look at how they are performing in roles such as prescribing (RPS 2016). The competency framework for prescribing practice can be used by district nurse prescribers to underpin the professional responsibility for prescribing practice (RPS 2016). The NMC (2018) has adopted this framework and dictates that this is the standard used to inform prescribing education programmes, and therefore it is useful to continue to use this framework on which to build your competence as a prescriber in practice.

The *Competency Framework for All Prescribers* (RPS 2016) depicts a person-centred approach to prescribing practice. It is compiled of ten competencies that are split into two domains – the consultation, and prescribing governance (See Table 3.1). The ten competency statements provide a framework to underpin prescribing practice and safe and effective decision making.

Box 3.2 – Various mnemonics that the prescriber may find useful

EASE

E   How **effective** is the product?
A   Is it **appropriate** for this person?
S   How **safe** is it?
E   Is the prescription cost-**effective**?

SIT DOWN SIR

S   Site or location of a sign/symptom
I   Intensity or severity
T   Type or nature
D   Duration
O   Onset
W   With (other symptoms)
N   Annoyed or aggravated by
S   Spread or radiation
I   Incidence or frequency
R   Relieved by

ASMETHOD

A   Age/appearance
S   Self or someone else
M   Medication
E   Extra medicines
T   Time persisting
H   History
O   Other symptoms
D   Danger symptoms

WWHAM

W   Who is the patient?
W   What are the symptoms?
H   How long have the symptoms been present?
A   Action taken
M   Medication being taken

Table 3.1 – The Competency Framework for All Prescribers

Consultation	Prescribing Governance
1. Assess patient 2. Consider the options 3. Come to a shared decision 4. Prescribe 5. Provide information 6. Monitor and review	7. Prescribe safely 8. Prescribe professionally 9. Improve prescribing practice 10. Prescribe as a part of a team

Source: Based on RPS (2016).

The Consultation

1. **Assess the patient**

   Use your usual nursing skills and the assessment model you are familiar with to assess your patient. You may also use a framework for holistic patient assessment that is used within your organisation.

2. **Consider the options**

   What options are available to you? For example, this may be to prescribe, to de-prescribe, to not prescribe, to offer advice, to refer on or to review at an agreed time. It may also be to direct the patient to over-the-counter remedies or lifestyle advice.

3. **Reach a shared decision**

   It is paramount to reach a decision in collaboration and agreement with your patient. This may take time to explore the options available, but it is essential for medicines optimisation and safe and effective prescribing practice.

4. **Prescribe**

   This may be the act of prescribing, de-prescribing or not prescribing. This needs to be person-centred and you must consider the patient when considering what you are prescribing, e.g. will they be able to swallow it? Do they have the dexterity to manage this medication? Do you need to ensure further support for the patient?

5. **Provide information**

   This is essential and refers to the information you need to give your patient not only on why you reached your prescribing decision, but also on the medicine itself, if the decision is to prescribe. You will need to inform the patient about how and when to take the medicine and for how long, and any special considerations such as contraindications to note. You should also inform the patient about the pharmacological action of the medication, about what side effects may be experienced and about safety netting, i.e. where to go and who to contact should they experience any worsening symptoms or problems.

6. **Monitor and review**

   You should ensure that you follow up and review your patient to ensure that the presenting complaint has been successfully dealt with and that no further problems have been experienced.

Prescribing Governance

7. **Prescribe safely**

   You should ensure that your prescribing decision is communicated to the wider integrated care team. This allows for safe decisions to be made subsequently and for an audit trail of practice should the patient experience any adverse outcomes.

   You should only ever prescribe within your scope of prescribing practice and utilise an evidence-based approach to your prescribing decision making.

8. **Prescribe professionally**

   You should only prescribe within your scope of prescribing practice and within the limitations of your role and NMC code (NMC 2019). You should discuss any prescribing decisions fully with the patient and their GP.

9. **Improve prescribing practice**

   You should reflect on your prescribing practice and consider how you can develop and enhance this for patients. You should undertake a review of your prescribing practice at least annually and ensure that you have an ongoing continuing professional development plan to remain up to date.

10. **Prescribe as part of a team**

    Remember that you are never prescribing in isolation. You are part of a wider and integrated team and have a plethora of resources available to support your decision making, and it is your responsibility as a district nurse prescriber to access these to ensure safe and effective prescribing practice.

Principles of Good Prescribing

A predecessor to the competency framework for all prescribers (RPS 2016) was the prescribing pyramid. Developed by the National Prescribing Centre in 1999, this is now incorporated by NICE. Although now superseded, the prescribing pyramid also offers a useable framework on which to base your prescribing decisions to ensure safe and effective patient-centred practice.

1. **Consider the patient**

   Who is the patient? Are they within your scope of prescribing practice? Who is the prescription for? Is the patient trying to access one for someone else or for future use? What is the presenting complaint, how long have they experienced it, are there any exacerbating or relieving interventions? What actions has the patient taken so far and what other medicines are being taken? What co-morbidities does the patient have? This is where your holistic assessment and use of mnemonics may come in useful.

2. **Which strategy?**

   Have you been able to establish a diagnosis on which to base your prescribing decision? Do you need to refer on to another prescriber or practitioner? Is a prescription needed at all? Is a prescription expected? Consider how you may manage this in practice. Only ever prescribe when there is a genuine need.

3. **Choice of product**

   You will need to ensure you take a patient-centred approach to choosing the product to prescribe; there is no point prescribing if the patient is unable to take the medication. You need to consider cost-efficacy in your selection of a product, and what is available to you within your local formulary.

4. **Negotiate a contract**

   You will need to ensure that a shared decision is made between you and your patient. If the patient is not involved or engaged in the decision-making process, the likelihood of them using the medicine effectively is much reduced. Shared decision-making also includes the provision of information to the patient and ensuring their understanding so that an informed decision is reached. The World Health Organization offers some decision-making aids online that can be used with patients when making decisions around medicines and interventions and can be useful in practice.

5. **Review**

   You should always ensure that you have provided safety netting information to your patient on what should they do and who to contact if symptoms persist, if symptoms worsen or if they become more acutely unwell. You should always ensure that you undertake a timely review of your prescribing decision to ensure patient safety and the efficacy of your decision making.

6. **Record-keeping**

   You should always document your prescribing decision making, as with any intervention you make, concurrent with the NMC code (NMC 2019). As previously discussed, you need to communicate your prescribing decision to all those involved in the patient's care, as subsequent decisions will be informed by what you have done. In addition, there must be an audit trail of what has been prescribed for the patient should they experience any unintentional adverse outcomes.

7. **Reflect**

   Reflecting on your prescribing practice and decision making will allow you to develop your knowledge and skills and to grow in confidence and competence as a prescriber. This will also help you develop the scope of your prescribing practice should you move into prescribing for other disease

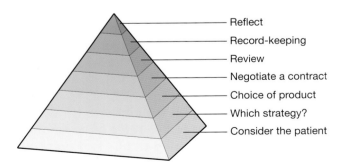

Figure 3.2 – The prescribing pyramid
Source: NPC (1999).

pathologies. Using supplementary prescribing and clinical management plans may also help you do this (see **Chapter 9** for more information). You will be able to share learning with others to ensure patient safety.

The Use of Information Technology (IT) Systems in Prescribing Decisions

There are a number of information technology (IT) systems available in primary care that support decision making. These can help by providing information on interactions and patient data. You may not have access to these as a district nurse and when you are out in the community undertaking home visits. You may be able to access some online resources remotely on mobile devices; however, these cannot always be depended on due to access issues and device malfunction. If you are unable to access the information you need, then you should delay your prescribing decision. Access to an up-to-date paper BNF will be useful to you in practice as you commence prescribing.

Reviewing your ePACT data regularly will help inform your prescribing practice, as it will help you identify trends on which you may wish to reflect and develop. Refer to **Chapter 7** for further information.

Turn to **Chapter 9** for more on the legal and ethical aspects of prescribing, and to **Chapter 10** to read more about the public health issues of prescribing.

Turn to **Chapter 12** for more information about personal reflection and professional development.

Conclusion

As you develop and become more adept in your prescribing role, you will need to make a variety of decisions. This chapter has explored the importance of thinking critically and considering human factors prior to making decisions. There are numerous decision-making models that have been proposed to try and assist nurses to make effective decisions. The use of mnemonics may assist you when gathering data in order that your prescribing decision is of the highest quality and is the best it can be for each patient.

Key Points of This Chapter

♦ Thinking critically is crucial to the decision-making process.

♦ There are numerous decision-making models that have been developed. It is worthwhile reading widely and finding one or two that suit you, both professionally and personally.

♦ At times, you may need to escalate concerns using a structured approach.

♦ The use of mnemonics may help you collect the data you need for improved decision making in your prescribing practice.

References and Further Reading

Aviation Safety Network (2018) Air accident statistics. Available at: https://aviation-safety.net/statistics/ (last accessed 6 June 2019).

Banning, M. (2008) A review of clinical decision making: Models and current research. *Journal of Clinical Nursing* 17(2): 187–195.

Benner, P. and Tanner, C. (1987) Clinical judgement: How expert nurses use intuition. *American Journal of Nursing* 87(1): 23–34.

Besco, R. (1999) PACE: Probe, Alert, Challenge and Emergency Action. *Business and Commercial Aviation* 84(6): 72–74.

British Medical Association (BMA) (2019) Dealing with the pharmaceutical industry. Available at: https://www.bma.org.uk/advice/career/studying-medicine/common-challenges-while-studying/dealing-with-the-pharmaceutical-industry (last accessed 24 July 2019).

British National Formulary (BNF). (2019) *BNF 78. September 2019 to March 2020.* London: Joint Formulary Committee.

Cioffi, J. (1997) Heuristics, servants to intuition, in clinical decision-making. *Journal of Advanced Nursing* 26: 203–208.

Clinical Human Factors Group (2018) Website. Available at: https://chfg.org (accessed 2 December 2019).

Department of Health and Social Care (DHSC) (2017) NHS becomes first healthcare system in the world to publish numbers of avoidable deaths. Available at: https://www.gov.uk/government/news/nhs-becomes-first-healthcare-system-in-the-world-to-publish-numbers-of-avoidable-deaths (last accessed 6 June 2019).

Elstein, A. S. and Schwarz, A. (2002) Clinical problem solving and diagnostic decision making: Selective review of the cognitive literature. *British Medical Journal* 423(7339): 729–732.

Facione, P. A. (2006) Critical thinking. What is it and why it counts. Available at: https://www.insightassessment.com/content/download/1176/7580/file/what&why.pdf (last accessed 6 June 2019).

Ford, S. (2015) Communication errors behind a third of hospital complaints. Available at: https://www.nursingtimes.net/roles/nurse-managers/communication-errors-behind-third-of-hospital-complaints/5090545.article (last accessed 24 July 2019).

Gambrill, E. (2012) *Critical Thinking in Clinical Practice*. 3rd edn. Hoboken, NJ: John Wiley.

General Medical Council (GMC) (2013) Good practice in prescribing and managing medical devices. Available at: https://www.gmc-uk.org/-/media/documents/Prescribing_guidance.pdf_59055247.pdf (last accessed 6 August 2019).

Hamm, R. M. (1988) Clinical intuition and clinical analysis: Expertise and the cognitive continuum. In J. Dowie and A. Eisten (eds), *Professional Judgement: A Reader in Clinical Decision Making*. Cambridge: Cambridge University Press, pp. 78–105.

Hammond, K., Stewart, T. R., Brehmer, B. et al. (1975) *Social Judgement Theory. Human Judgement and Decision Processes*. New York: Academic Press.

Hammond, K. R. (2000) *Judgement Under Stress*. New York. Oxford University Press.

Ignatavicius, D. (2001) Critical thinking skills for the bedside nurse. *Nursing Management* 32(1): 37–39.

Johansen M. L. and O'Brien J. L. (2015) Decision making in nursing practice. *Nursing Forum* 51(1): 40–48.

Kahneman, D. (2011) *Thinking Fast and Slow*. London: Penguin.

King, L. and Clark, J. M. (2002) Intuition and the development of expertise in surgical ward and intensive care nurses. *Journal of Advanced Nursing* 37(4): 322–329.

Manias, E., Aiken, R. and Dunning, T. (2004) Decision-making models used by 'graduate nurses' managing patients' medications. *Journal of Advanced Nursing* 47(3): 270–278.

Marquis, B. and Huston, C. (2017) *Leadership Roles and Management Functions in Nursing: Theory and Application*. 9th edn. Philadelphia, PA: Lippincott Williams and Wilkins.

Matthews, C. (2018) Human factors affecting paramedic practice. In A. Y. Blaber (ed.), *Blaber's Foundations for Paramedic Practice. A Theoretical Perspective*. London. Open University Press. McGraw-Hill Education, pp. 75–88.

Muir, N. (2004) Clinical decision making: Theory and practice. *Nursing Standard* 18(36): 47–52.

National Institute for Health and Clinical Excellence (NICE) (2018) Website. Available at: https://www.nice.org.uk (last accessed 2 December 2019).

National Prescribing Centre (NPC) (1999) *Nurse Prescribing Bulletin. Signposts for Prescribing Nurses – General Principles of Good Prescribing*. London: National Prescribing Centre.

National Quality Board (NQB) (2013) Human factors in healthcare. A concordat from the National Quality Board. Available at: https://www.england.nhs.uk/wp-content/uploads/2013/11/nqb-hum-fact-concord.pdf (last accessed 6 June 2019).

Nursing and Midwifery Council (NMC) (2018) *Realising Professionalism: Standards for Education and Training. Part 3: Standards for Prescribing Programmes*. London: Nursing and Midwifery Council.

Nursing and Midwifery Council (NMC) (2019) The code. Available at: https://www.nmc.org.uk/standards/code/read-the-code-online/ (last accessed 28 January 2020).

O'Neill, E. S. and Dluhy, N. M. (1997) A longitudinal framework for fostering critical thinking and diagnostic reasoning. *Journal of Advanced Nursing* 26(4): 825–832.

O'Neill, E. S., Dluhy, N. M. and Chin, E. (2005) Modelling novice clinical reasoning for a computerised decision support system. *Journal of Advanced Nursing* 49(1): 68–71.

Pritchard, M. J. (2006) Professional development. Making effective clinical decisions: a framework for nurse practitioners. *British Journal of Nursing* 15(3): 128–130.

Reason J. (2000) Human error: Models and management. *British Medical Journal* 320(7237): 768–770.

Riem, N., Boet, S., Bould, M. et al. (2012) Do technical skills correlate with non-technical skills in crisis resource management? A simulation study. *British Journal of Anesthesia* 109(5): 723–728.

Royal College of Nursing (RCN) (2017) Teamwork. Available at: https://www.rcn.org.uk/clinical-topics/patient-safety-and-human-factors (last accessed 6 June 2019).

Royal Pharmaceutical Society (RPS) (2016) *A Competency Framework for All Prescribers.* London: The Royal Pharmaceutical Society.

Simon, H. A. (1959) Theories of decision-making in economics and behavioral science. *American Economic Review* 49: 253–283.

Tanner, C. A., Padrick, K. P., Westfall, U. E. et al. (1987) Diagnostic reasoning strategies of nurses and nursing students. *Nursing Research* 36(6): 358–365.

Tversky, A. and Kahneman, D. (1982) Judgments of and by representativeness. In D. Kahneman, P. Slovic and A. Tversky (eds), *Judgment under Uncertainty: Heuristics and Biases.* Cambridge: Cambridge University Press, pp. 84–100.

Chapter 4
Basic Pharmacology

Jennifer Gorman

In This Chapter

- ♦ Introduction
- ♦ Key terminology
- ♦ Drug design and delivery
- ♦ Pharmacodynamics
- ♦ Pharmacokinetics
- ♦ Dose response and steady state
- ♦ Conclusion
- ♦ Key points of this chapter
- ♦ References and further reading
- ♦ Useful websites.

Introduction

As a prescriber, you need to understand pharmacology; that is, how drugs interact with the body. This includes the mechanisms by which drugs produce a response, as well as how they are processed and eventually removed by the body. At a basic level, we can think of pharmacology as the journey of a medicine through the body. For example, if a tablet is swallowed, how does the drug actually get to where it needs to go at the concentration needed to produce a therapeutic response? When it gets there, how does the drug produce a response at a cellular level and why is this important? Once it has done its job, how is the drug processed and then removed by the body?

There are formularies and guidelines that have an important role in clinical decision making, but in practice patients are often not straightforward. They may be prescribed multiple medicines for a range of co-morbidities or perhaps have a condition that changes how drugs are processed, as in renal impairment. Understanding how these medicines interact with the body and each other is fundamental in supporting effective clinical decision making in these patients.

The aim of this chapter is to give you a grounding in the basics of the topic. It begins by giving an overview of pharmacology and considering how drugs are designed and developed. This is followed by sections on the two main branches of the discipline: pharmacodynamics and pharmacokinetics. Examples are given using a range of commonly used drugs to link the concepts covered to clinical practice. The aim is that you will then be able to apply the concepts included in this chapter to any drug within your scope of practice, supporting safe and effective prescribing.

Key Terminology

It is likely that readers of this book will have differing levels of background knowledge of pharmacology, but even if you have some knowledge, the information can act as a refresher.

The summary of key terminology is given below to allow you to reflect on your existing knowledge. Are these terms you have heard before? Sometimes terms like 'efficacy' and 'potency' get used, but it is clear that they have not been fully understood. Take a minute to consider your own understanding.

If you feel that you know nothing and the summary in Table 4.1 makes no sense yet, do not worry – we cover all these terms in this chapter.

Table 4.1 – Summary of key pharmacology terms

Term	Definition
Affinity	The tendency for a drug to bind to a receptor
Agonist	A drug that **activates** the activity of a receptor, producing a change in a physiological system
Antagonist	A drug that **inhibits** the activity of a receptor by blocking the production of a response by an agonist
Bioavailability	The fraction or percentage of drug that reaches the systemic circulation unchanged
Bioequivalence	Drug products that are formulated in a way that they are generally considered therapeutically interchangeable
Dose-response curve	The relationship between the dose of a drug and the pharmacological response

Table 4.1 – Summary of key pharmacology terms (*continued*)

Term	Definition
Drug target	The protein (or occasionally DNA, mRNA) that a drug binds to, producing a physiological effect. These proteins are often receptors (e.g. ion channels, enzymes or nuclear receptors)
Efficacy	The tendency for a drug to activate the receptor when bound
ED_{50}	The dose that produces 50% of the maximal response of a drug
E_{max}	The dose that produces the maximal response of a drug
Formulation	The process by which a medicinal product that can be administered to a patient is made from the active ingredient and other chemical compounds
Partial agonist	An agonist that produces a maximal response that is less than the maximal response produced by a full agonist
Pharmacodynamics	The field of study concerned with what drugs do to the body
Pharmacokinetics	The field of study concerned with what the body does to drugs
Potency	The concentration of drug needed to produce a defined level of response
Specificity	How selectively a drug will bind to a particular receptor
$T_{1/2}$ (Drug half-live)	The time taken for the concentration of drug to decrease to 50%
Volume of distribution (Vd)	The volume of plasma that would be necessary to account for the total amount of a drug in the patient's body if that drug were present throughout the body at the same concentration as found in the plasma

Drug Design and Delivery

Before concentrating on the more detailed aspects of pharmacology, it is worth considering a few basic principles of drug design and delivery.

A good place to start this is by defining pharmacology.

Pharmacology is:

'The study of the effects of drugs on the function of living systems'.
(Rang et al. 2016, p. 25)

Humans have known for a long time that compounds can be used to produce an effect on living systems. The Greeks and Romans wrote pharmacopeias listing the uses of many herbal compounds. Until relatively recently, the main way in which treatments were assessed was empirically – observing what effect a treatment had following administration. There was, however, a lack of understanding of how exactly the treatment achieved its therapeutic effect.

Modern pharmacology focuses on understanding how drugs work at a physiological level, meaning that drugs can be targeted specifically and designed to optimise therapeutic outcomes (see **Box 4.2**). The key elements of pharmacology are stated in **Box 4.1**. Importantly, this understanding also helps to minimise toxicity and side effects.

Box 4.1 – Key elements of pharmacology

♦ The study of the chemical constitution of drugs
♦ The study of the effects of drugs on cells and tissues
♦ The study of the therapeutic use of drugs to treat illness and disease.

Box 4.2 – An example of how modern pharmacology can be used to optimise therapeutic outcomes

Opioids act on targets in the body that produce analgesia and have been used for centuries for that purpose. However, they do not act specifically on the targets linked to pain and so produce side effects, such as constipation and respiratory depression. Modern synthetic opioid-based drugs, such as tramadol and fentanyl, have been developed so that they act more specifically on the receptors linked to analgesia

This has been achieved through:
♦ Knowledge of the chemical structure of the drugs
♦ Knowledge of how the drug acts to produce an analgesic response
♦ Knowledge of other body systems and how they are affected by the drug.

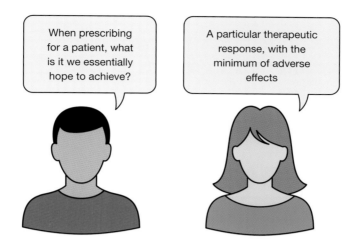

Is it a Drug or a Medicine?

We tend to use the terms 'drug' and 'medicine' interchangeably, but in this section we will briefly consider what the differences are between the two. Whilst in practice such semantics may not seem particularly significant, understanding how drugs are 'packaged' into medicines is important in terms of understanding how they ultimately produce a pharmacological affect.

A **drug** is a chemical, other than a nutrient, that produces a biological response in a living organism. However, a biological response does not necessarily correspond to a therapeutic response. This means that poisons are drugs, but we wouldn't usually give these to our patients. Even drugs that can be used therapeutically can lead to a response that we don't want if they are taken at too high a dose.

A **medicine** is a preparation that contains a drug at a dose that will produce a therapeutic response. It usually also contains other chemicals that are included for various reasons, such as to make it easier to administer or store. So, it contains a therapeutic level of drug, but it will almost always contain other ingredients too.

The process of making a drug into a medicine that can be administered to a patient is called 'formulation'. There are different types of medicinal products, which include the same drug in different formulations (see Box 4.3 for an example). Many drugs are available in a variety of formulations that can be selected depending on the patient's needs. Always remember that the 'package' in which the drug comes can mean that it has slightly different pharmacological properties. We will discuss some of the implications of formulation in the pharmacokinetics section on routes of administration.

There are many ingredients that can be used in formulating medicines to help make them suitable for patients to use. A few examples you may see listed in the Summary of Product Characteristics (SPC) are listed in Table 4.2.

Box 4.3 – An example of formulations of paracetamol that are available

♦ Tablet
♦ Capsule
♦ Dispersible tablet
♦ IV solution
♦ Oral solution
♦ Suppositories.

Table 4.2 – Examples of some of the types of ingredients used in formulation

Ingredient	Purpose
Excipient	Pharmacologically inactive substances, which can be used for a wide range of purposes – for example, as a bulking agent in tablets or coating for modified release preparations
Stabiliser	To physically and chemically stabilise drugs so that they do not break down during manufacture and storage
Solvent	A substance that can dissolve a drug so it can be made into a solution

Pharmacodynamics

The human body is an amazingly complex biological structure with a vast network of mechanisms that control its physiological functions. As we saw in the previous section, drugs are designed to interact with these mechanisms in order to produce a response. However, the complexity of the body means that no drug works entirely selectively to produce only the intended therapeutic response. This is one of the challenges when developing new drugs, as there can be unexpected consequences when drugs begin to be used *in vivo* that have not been encountered during *in vitro* testing. In this section, we will consider how drugs interact with the body to produce a response and will introduce pharmacological principles that are important to consider when prescribing.

Definition: Pharmacodynamics: what the drug does to the body

Mechanisms of Drug Action

Drugs interact with targets in the human body to produce their responses. These targets are often receptors on or inside cells, and so the term drug–receptor interaction is often used to describe these interactions; see Box 4.4.

Box 4.4 – Examples of physiological responses that can be produced through drug–receptor interactions

- Change in the contractility of a tissue, e.g. muscle
- Change in excitability of neurons and thus neural stimulation
- Changes in gene transcription.

The extent of change caused by the drug depends on both its **affinity** and **efficacy**.

Drug–Receptor Interactions

As Figure 4.1 shows, the shape of the drug and the target is predominantly what defines whether the drug binds to the receptor and produces a response. In drug development there is a significant amount of work which goes into designing and then refining the chemical structure to optimise the shape to get the best possible fit.

These interactions are often described using the lock and key hypothesis, and we can imagine this like the shape of a key used to open a lock. The key is made up of a whole range of cuts and groves, giving it a unique 3D shape. Other keys might fit partially into the lock, but it is only the one shape that will open it fully.

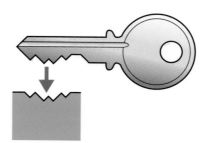

Figure 4.1 – Diagram showing the 'lock and key' hypothesis

Drugs are designed to take advantage of this principle, either by binding to activate the receptor or instead occupying the receptor binding site to prevent the binding of endogenous chemicals:

- Drugs that are designed to fit the lock and activate a physiological process are known as **agonists**.
- Drugs that are designed to block the lock from binding chemicals that can activate them are known as **antagonists** (see Figure 4.2).

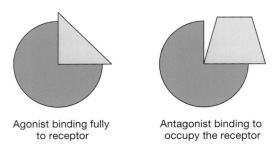

Agonist binding fully
to receptor

Antagonist binding to
occupy the receptor

Figure 4.2 – Diagram showing differences between agonist and antagonist binding

For example, antihistamines are antagonists that attach to histamine receptors, blocking endogenous histamine from causing an allergic reaction.

Affinity, Efficacy, Specificity and Potency

These terms are often used interchangeably yet they represent very different pharmacological concepts. Before looking at the other types of drug interactions it is worth focusing in more detail on these terms to make sure they are clear.

Affinity is the tendency for a drug to bind to a receptor. It can be thought of in basic terms of how attracted the molecule is to the receptor binding site. Thinking of an example, we may have two drugs, both of which produce an equal response when bound to a receptor, but one is much more strongly attracted than the other to this receptor. The one that is more strongly attracted is said to have a higher affinity for the drug target and it is likely this one will produce a greater effect *in vivo* because it will bind much more readily with the target.

Efficacy is the tendency of the drug to produce a response when bound to a receptor. As we have seen, the shape of the drug and the receptor play a key role in this. A drug may have a high affinity for a receptor but have no efficacy, so it really wants to bind with the receptor but produces no response when it does. These in fact are generally the key characteristics of an antagonist – high affinity but no efficacy. Conversely, what we are usually aiming for with an agonist is a high affinity and a high efficacy.

Specificity is a term that describes how selectively a drug binds to a particular receptor. It is important to realise that in the body there are a whole host of structurally similar receptors that regulate quite different physiological responses. Often drugs will bind to more than one receptor subtype. These receptors can also be spread throughout different tissues in the body. For example, Beta-1 receptors are found in the cardiac tissue and beta-blockers such as atenolol bind to these receptors to produce their therapeutic effect. They can also bind to some degree to Beta-2 receptors found in the bronchioles, causing bronchoconstriction. This causes complications in asthma and it is lack of selectivity that is the reason that beta-blockers should not be used in this group of patients. We can see then that ideally a drug will have a high level of specificity as this will reduce the likelihood of side effects. Interestingly, however, the lack of specificity of some drugs has led to them being used for other indications than those they were originally licensed for.

Potency refers to the amount of drug required to produce a defined level of response. If for example 1 milligram of Drug A produces the same response as 10 milligrams of Drug B, then we can see that Drug A is more potent. This does not mean it is 'stronger' per se, but merely that you need less drug to produce a particular therapeutic response. In practice you may hear patients saying that they have been prescribed a 'stronger' medicine—for example, if their new medication for treating hypertension is a 500 milligram tablet, whereas the previous medication was a 100 milligram tablet. Because of variations in potency, it does not follow that the new medication will cause a reduction in blood pressure that is five times greater.

Other Types of Drug–Receptor Interactions

Whilst agonists and antagonists are the most common types of drug–receptor interactions, it is important to be aware that there are several others.

Partial Agonists

As the name suggests, these drugs bind to receptors, leading to partial activation of a physiological response. This may be useful when it is necessary to produce a smaller response than a full agonist would.

For example, buprenorphine is a partial agonist of μ-opioid receptors and one of its uses is supporting opioid-dependent patients when withdrawing from opioids. When administered, it produces a response, but, as the graph in Figure 4.3 shows, not of the same magnitude as opioids such as heroin that are full agonists of μ-opioid receptors.

As a partial agonist, the maximum effect of an equivalent dose of buprenorphine is less than that of a full agonist such as morphine or heroin.

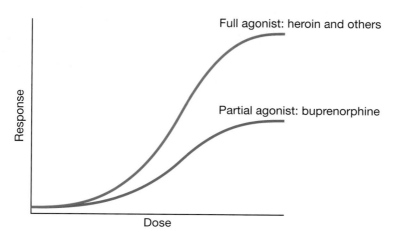

Figure 4.3 – Graph showing effect of buprenorphine as a partial agonist versus heroin

Competitive and Non-competitive Antagonists

Competitive antagonists compete with other agents to occupy receptor binding sites. The two-way arrow in Figure 4.4 highlights that this is a reversible effect and depends on the affinity that both the agonist and antagonist have for the receptor binding site. Some drugs, such as naloxone, can displace other molecules from the receptor binding site, as illustrated in Figure 4.4. Other competitive antagonists merely compete with other molecules to occupy the binding site.

Naloxone is a competitive antagonist that acts to displace both agonists and partial agonists at opioid receptors. It has essentially no pharmacological activity in the absence of opioids and is used to treat an opioid overdose.

Non-competitive antagonists are different in that they bind irreversibly to the receptor binding site, as illustrated in Figure 4.5. This means that the only way for the effect of the antagonist to be overcome is when the receptor itself is broken down and replaced.

For example, aspirin is a non-competitive antagonist. Its use as an antiplatelet for chronic prophylaxis is due to irreversible binding to receptors on platelets.

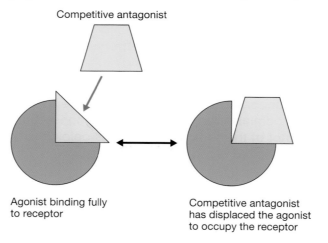

Competitive antagonist

Agonist binding fully
to receptor

Competitive antagonist
has displaced the agonist
to occupy the receptor

Figure 4.4 – Diagram showing action of competitive antagonists

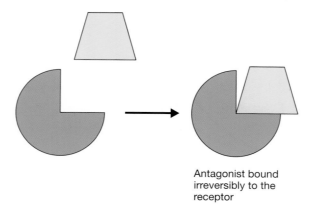

Antagonist bound
irreversibly to the
receptor

Figure 4.5 – Diagram showing action of non-competitive antagonists

Platelets have a lifespan of ten days, which could potentially lead to problems with the effect lasting the lifetime of the platelet. However, the risk is minimised as only low doses are used for this indication and because platelets are replenished from the bone marrow daily.

Inverse Agonists

Drugs known as inverse agonists produce a net decrease in the basal activity of the receptor with which they interact. To understand this concept, we must first understand the concept of a two-state model of receptors. This model suggests that receptors exist in two different conformational states, effectively meaning they exist in two different 3D shapes. One shape is a resting state where the receptor is essentially inactive. The shape, however, changes when the receptor is active and able to produce a response, as **Figure 4.6** shows. Normally they exist in an equilibrium between the two states.

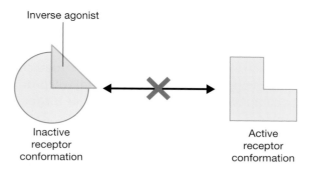

Figure 4.6 – Diagram showing action of inverse agonist, two-state model

An inverse agonist has a greater affinity for the resting state of the receptor and so binds more readily to the receptor in this state. Once the inverse agonist is bound to the receptor, it is unable to change into the active conformation, causing the equilibrium between active and inactive to shift in favour of the inactive. The net effect is to reduce the number of active receptors, thus causing an overall decrease in the basal physiological activity.

Allosteric Interactions

Allosteric sites are secondary binding sites on receptors that can change the affinity of molecules for the primary binding site, as can be seen in **Figure 4.7**. They do this by causing the shape of the binding site to change. This can mean that other molecules may either be more or less likely to bind and cause a response.

An example of this is the drug cinnacalet (brand name Mimpara). This drug is licensed for treatment of hyperparathyroidism and works by binding to an allosteric site on the calcium sensing receptor on the surface of the chief cell of the parathyroid gland. This causes the receptor to have increased sensitivity to extracellular calcium, which consequently leads to a reduction in circulating parathyroid hormone.

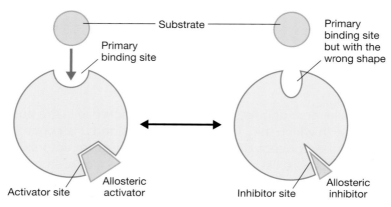

Figure 4.7 – Diagram showing allosteric interactions

For more information, see the SPC at: https://www.medicines.org.uk/emc/product/5599#.

Types of Drug Targets

As we have already discussed, the purpose of giving a medication to a patient is to produce some kind of physiological response that will produce a therapeutic outcome. In this section, we will look at the types of targets that we can use to produce a response.

Ligand-gated Ion Channels

Physiological processes are regulated in a variety of ways, one of which is by the movement of ions (charged particles) across a cell membrane. The movement of ions is regulated using transmembrane channels that allow the selective passage of ions, such as Na^+, K^+ and Cl^-, into and out of cells. They open and close in response to the binding of a chemical messenger or ligand. Ligands can be drugs, which either activate or inhibit opening of the channels by binding directly to the channel or an intermediary receptor. Ion channels tend to regulate processes that are linked to rapid physiological changes (see **Figure 4.8**), e.g. the regulation of the heartbeat or the conduction of impulses through neurons.

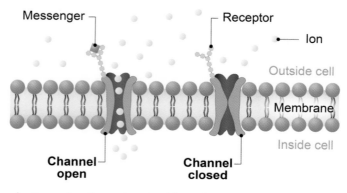

Figure 4.8 – Action of a ligand-gated ion channel
Source: designua / 123RF.

For example:

♦ **Local anaesthetics**: block sodium (Na⁺) channels in pain neurons. This stops sodium entering the cell on which conduction of the nerve impulse to pain sensors in the brain depends. This means that conduction of pain signals is halted and the brain does not perceive the pain signal.
♦ **Nifedipine**: blocks receptors on calcium channels in arterioles, hence it is in the class of drugs that are known as calcium channel blockers.
♦ **Benzodiazepines**: act on inhibitory GABA receptors found on neurons in the central nervous system. They open chloride (Cl⁻) channels that are linked to the receptors and allow movement of chloride out of the cells. This potentiates the inhibitory effect of the neuron and is the reason that benzodiazepines are used to manage seizures.

G-protein-coupled Receptors (GPCRs)

These receptors are coupled with proteins known as a G-proteins, which consist of seven transmembrane segments (see **Figure 4.9**) linked to intracellular G-proteins. They conduct signals through their coupling with intracellular

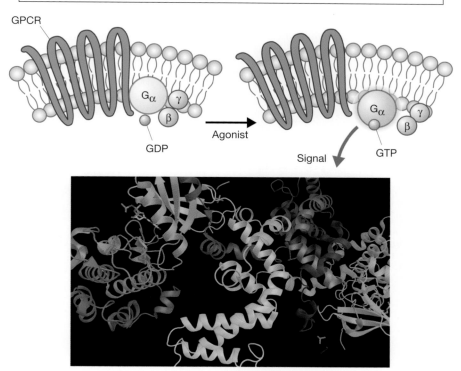

GTP: Guanosine triphosphate	β: G-protein β subunit
GDP: Guanosine diphosphate	γ: G-protein γ subunit
Gα: G-protein α subunit	

Figure 4.9 – Diagram showing action of GPCRs and a 3D image of the structure of a GPCR, Kinase 6
Source: A. © Class Professional Publishing B. Iculig / 123RF.

systems. Extracellular binding therefore activates a cascade that leads to a change in intracellular processes. These receptors are widely spread through the body and act to regulate a whole host of physiological responses. Examples that you may be familiar with in this family include opioid, dopamine and 5-HT receptors. Drugs acting on these receptors also produce a relatively rapid response, but because of the time taken to transduce the signal, the response is slower than is the case for drugs acting on ion channels.

Enzyme-coupled Receptors

Enzymes are large complex proteins whose function in the body is to catalyse a range of reactions that are involved in regulating a whole host of different physiological processes. Drugs that bind to receptors coupled to these receptors can therefore alter these processes. As with GPCRs, the enzyme is involved in conducting a signal intracellularly. However, the way in which the signal is conducted by the enzyme is different from the GPCR (see **Figure 4.10**). In its

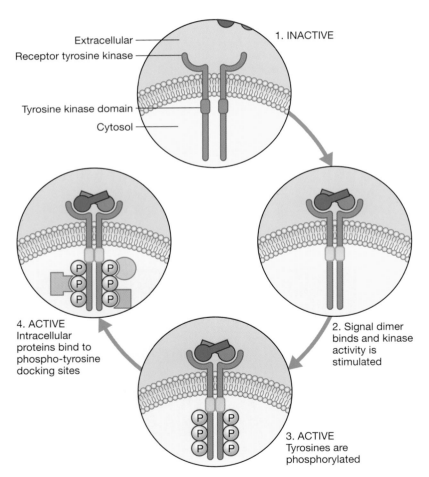

Figure 4.10 – Diagram showing how enzyme-couple receptors work, using the example of tyrosine kinase receptors

inactive state, the enzyme consists of two separate molecules. Binding of a ligand, such as a drug or a hormone, to an extracellular binding site causes the separate intracellular kinase domain to associate. This leads to phosphorylation of the intracellular kinase, which allows these to act as docking sites for other intracellular proteins. This ultimately leads to a cellular response.

For example, aspirin binds to the enzyme cyclooxygenase (COX), inhibiting its ability to catalyse the synthesis of prostaglandins. It is this interaction that produces its anti-inflammatory, analgesic and antipyretic action.

Nuclear or Intracellular Receptors

These receptors are found within the cell and exist unbound either in the cytoplasm or the nucleus. Those that exist in the cytoplasm move within the nucleus after binding with a ligand, as they require access to DNA to produce their response. When activated, they cause changes in gene expression and therefore protein synthesis (see **Figure 4.11**). Because of this, it can take hours or days to see a response.

Examples of nuclear or intracellular receptors include hormones such as testosterone and oestrogen, as well as glucocorticoid steroids.

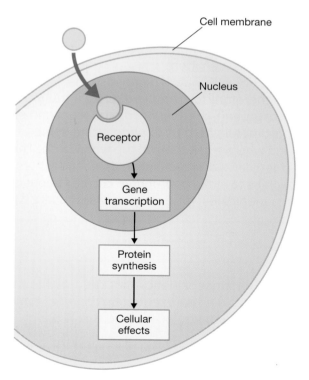

Figure 4.11 – Diagram showing action of nuclear or intracellular receptors

Self-test exercise:

♦ What is the difference between affinity and efficacy?
♦ What pharmacological and biological properties lead drugs to cause side effects?
♦ How do dose and response differ between full, partial and inverse agonists, as well as antagonists?
♦ What are the main types of drug targets?

Finally, think about some of the drugs you will be prescribing and spend some time looking at their pharmacodynamic properties. You can find this information at: https://www.medicines.org.uk/emc. Use the search function to look up drugs relevant to your practice. When you click on the monograph for a drug, you will see it is split into different sections, one of which is the pharmacodynamic properties of that medicine.

Pharmacokinetics

Pharmacokinetics helps describe the journey of the drug into, around and then out of the body. It is concerned with what the body does to the drug, as opposed to pharmacodynamics where the focus is on what therapeutic response is produced in the body. Essentially, when a medicine is administered to a patient, it must be absorbed by the body and it must then be distributed around the body to the tissue where it will produce a response. Once in the body it will be broken down through metabolism and finally eliminated from the body. There are therefore four key elements in the journey of medicines through the body: absorption, distribution, metabolism and elimination. These pharmacokinetic parameters help us to understand some of the key features about medicines and why we use them in the way we do. They can help us to explain why some medicines are taken once daily and others four times a day. They can also support us to make appropriate choices about the route by which we give our patients medicines, for example, when to use IV instead of oral.

Definition: Pharmacokinetics: what the body does to the drug

The four key areas of pharmacokinetics that are used to characterise what happens to the drug *in vivo* are represented by the mnemonic ADME. This will help you remember these four key areas (see Box 4.5).

Box 4.5 – ADME

Absorption   Distribution   Metabolism   Elimination

Absorption of Drugs into the Body

The process of a drug moving from site of administration into the systemic circulation is known as absorption. The complexity of this process depends on the route of administration. For example, absorption of drugs given orally depends on the drug not being degraded in the gastrointestinal (GI) tract, as well as the ability to cross the intestinal epithelium. Drugs given intravenously bypass these problems. In this section, we will look at the physiological and physicochemical factors that are important in absorption.

General Considerations

The rate and extent of absorption depends on a number of factors and is influenced by how medicines are formulated and the route of administration chosen (see Box 4.6 for details).

Routes of Administration

There are a whole range of routes by which drugs can be administered, all of which have their own pros and cons. There are three broad categories into which all the routes of administration can be divided:

♦ Enteral: This route includes anything that is absorbed into the systemic circulation via the GI tract. Mainly this will be via ingestion orally, but it also includes patients with enteral feeding tubes such as PEGs.
♦ Parenteral: This route includes anything that is given directly into the body by means of an injection. IV, SC and IM are all parenteral routes of administration.
♦ Topical: This route includes anything that is applied to produce a local response. Usually this is applied to the skin, but can also include application to other tissues, such as eye, ear and nasal products. There are also some medicines available that are applied topically to the skin but whose effects are reliant on systemic absorption. These include transdermal patches.

For each of these, there are a range of factors that influence the rate and extent of absorption of different drugs.

Table 4.3 gives an overview of some of the important factors around the absorption of drugs via different routes of administration.

> ## Box 4.6 – Some factors affecting absorption
>
> ♦ The amount of blood perfusion there is to the site of absorption
> ♦ The surface area available over which absorption can take place
> ♦ The contact time of the drug with the site of absorption
> ♦ The chemical characteristics of the drug, e.g. how lipid or 'water-loving' it is (the terms lipophilic and hydrophilic are used to describe this), or how stable it is.

Table 4.3 – Some important factors in the absorption of drugs

Route	Factor	Examples
Oral	◆ The rate of gastric emptying ◆ Gastric motility ◆ The gastric pH, which can affect the stability of the drug and the extent of absorption ◆ Some drugs utilise active transport processes where the body actually actively absorbs the drug using pumps ◆ The size of the drug molecule ◆ The formulation given, e.g. tablet requires dissolution, liquid does not ◆ How soluble the drug is in the GI tract ◆ How lipophilic or hydrophilic the drug is.	This is the most common route of administration and most products are available orally. Note the variety of formulations available that manipulate physiological factors, e.g. modified release and enteric-coated medicines.
Intravenous	◆ This bypasses the need for absorption across a membrane, so IV drugs are rapidly absorbed ◆ Excipients must not cause irritation at injection site ◆ As this can result in high concentrations of drug at the site of administration, the speed of injection may need to be considered.	Vancomycin – when given orally, it is not absorbed in the GI tract and only has a local action.
Subcutaneous/ intramuscular	◆ Local perfusion of tissues and the site of injection can affect absorption ◆ Increased perfusion can cause more rapid absorption (e.g. following exercise) ◆ Decreased perfusion can slow absorption (e.g. heart failure) ◆ Formulation can be used to delay release of drugs, e.g. depot injections of drugs for mental health and contraception.	Paliperidone IM depot injection lasts three months due to low water solubility leading to slow absorption.

Table 4.3 – Some important factors in the absorption of drugs (*continued*)

Route	Factor	Examples
Topical	◆ Often used for local action ◆ Systemic absorption may occur and must be considered when prescribing ◆ For drugs that are being used for their systemic action, the epithelial and cutaneous tissues present a significant barrier to absorption ◆ Drugs must have low molecular weight and high lipid solubility for this route.	Steroid creams used in treating local inflammation. Eye drops and nasal sprays are considered topical, as applied to epithelial tissue.
Transdermal	◆ A form of topical administration where patches are formulated for sustained release of drug into the systemic circulation ◆ Skin is a significant barrier for drugs to cross ◆ Useful where consistent serum levels of the drug are required ◆ Only suitable for lipid soluble because of the lipid nature of the skin.	Opioid derivatives, e.g. fentanyl and buprenorphine; hormone patches.
Sublingual	◆ Allows fast absorption across the mucosal membrane of the mouth ◆ Useful when drugs are extensively metabolised by liver enzymes / unstable at gastric pH.	Glyceryl trinitrate; lorazepam tablets used off licence in acute anxiety to avoid parenteral administration.
Rectal	◆ Useful in patients where oral access is a problem, e.g. vomiting or Nil by Mouth ◆ Good absorption via this route and can minimise the effects of first pass metabolism (see explanation below) ◆ Can be used to achieve a local effect or a systemic effect.	Suppositories, enemas and foams all available.

(*continued*)

Table 4.3 – Some important factors in the absorption of drugs (*continued*)

Route	Factor	Examples
Inhalation	◆ Useful due to the large absorptive surface area in lungs ◆ Local administration for respiratory disease allows smaller doses to be used than via oral administration ◆ Mainly used for administration of locally acting drugs ◆ Some volatile gases (e.g. anaesthetics) are administered by this route.	Steroid inhalers; beta-agonist inhalers; gaseous anaesthetics

How Quickly Does Each Route Take to Work?
Table 4.4 shows how the rate of absorption can vary between different routes and result in variation in the onset of action for different formulations.

Table 4.4 – Rate of absorption and variations for the onset of action

Time of onset of action	Dosage forms
Seconds	Intravenous injections
Minutes	Intramuscular and subcutaneous injections, buccal tablets, aerosols, gases
Minutes to hours	Short-term depot injections, capsules, tablets, modified-release tablets, solutions, suspensions, powders, granules
Several hours	Enteric-coated formulations
Days to weeks	Depot injections, implants
Varies	Topical preparations

Source: Aulton and Taylor (2013).

Think about:

♦ What are the main pros and cons of each route of administration?
♦ Look at the factors that can affect absorption again and then think about how important they are for each different route.
♦ Consider the factors that might influence your decision on which route to use when prescribing a medication for managing pain.

First Pass Metabolism

Drugs can be metabolised before they even enter the circulation when blood from the small intestine travels via the hepatic portal vein to the liver, before then entering the systemic circulation.

This is known as first pass metabolism, and with some drugs the dose is metabolised significantly before it can reach the site of action (see **Box 4.7**). This means that there can be a large variation in the serum concentration resulting from a dose given parenterally versus when given orally.

Box 4.7 – Drugs that undergo extensive first pass metabolism

♦ Aspirin
♦ Glyceryl trinitrate
♦ Levodopa
♦ Morphine
♦ Metoprolol
♦ Salbutamol
♦ Verapamil.

Bioavailability and Area Under the Concentration Time Curve (AUC)

There are several factors that can affect the amount of drug that is absorbed into the systemic circulation. These include the first pass metabolism described above, along with others such as degradation in gastric acid or the barrier presented by the intestinal mucosa. Often, therefore, the full dose of a drug given orally does not reach the systemic circulation. This is in contrast with drugs given IV as they are introduced directly into the systemic circulation.

Bioavailability describes the fraction or percentage of drug that reaches the systemic circulation following oral administration. According to the SPC, amoxicillin capsules are approximately 70% bioavailable. This means that only 70% of the oral dose will reach the systemic circulation. The bioavailability of the IV injection will in contrast be 100%.

The AUC looks at the extent of absorption and elimination by sampling serum concentration over time in test subjects. The concentration points are then plotted on a graph against time which gives a curve as concentration rises following administration and then falls as elimination occurs. The resulting area underneath this graphical curve essentially shows the extent to which the drug has been present in the body. These curves are plotted separately following oral and IV administration, and the resulting figures are used to estimate bioavailability by dividing AUC_{oral} by $AUC_{intravenous}$. The AUC is something you may see included in the pharmacology section of a medicine's SPC.

> When switching between routes, there can be differences in absorption, which can be clinically significant, leading to a difference in bioavailability. This is the amount of a drug that reaches the systemic circulation unchanged.

There can also be variations in bioavailability when the same route is used but a different type of formulation, like a tablet or a liquid, is given. For example, Table 4.5 shows the different dose equivalents between citalopram tablets and oral solution.

Some drugs are in fact so prone to variations in bioavailability that even different makes of the same formulation, such as tablets, can show variation in bioavailability that can have a clinical impact. Patients stabilised on these medicines should therefore be prescribed their medication by brand. This is the case with several antiepileptic drugs; for example, guidance from the MHRA suggests that carbamazepine tablets must always be prescribed by brand or branded generic for epilepsy because of differences in bioavailability between formulations.

If, however, there is no clinical impact on substituting one formulation for another, then the formulations can be said to be **bioequivalent**.

Table 4.5 – Citalopram doses for different oral formulations

Tablet dose equivalent	Solution
10 milligrams	8 milligrams (4 drops)
20 milligrams	16 milligrams (8 drops)
30 milligrams	24 milligrams (12 drops)
30 milligrams	32 milligrams (16 drops)

Think about:

Is there a clinical difference between the different formulations of drug you will be prescribing?

♦ Can you name a drug that you know you must prescribe by brand?
♦ What factors can you think of that might affect the bioavailability of a medicine?
♦ Is there any monitoring you would need to do when switching between formulations?
♦ How would you explain to a patient why the dose of their medication has changed if you switch formulation and there is a dose adjustment (as in the case of citalopram liquid and tablets)?

Distribution

Once the drug has been absorbed, it is distributed around the body via the circulatory system. It is important to realise that this distribution will not be uniform due to the complex makeup of the body. In order to describe the distribution of drugs, we must imagine the body as made up of multiple compartments. The different composition of the compartments means that some drugs will naturally partition into some compartments rather than others, leading to variable drug concentrations in different compartments.

Distribution into Body Compartments

The body can be seen as consisting of five main compartments:

♦ Intracellular fluid
♦ Interstitial fluid
♦ Blood plasma
♦ Other bodily fluids (e.g. cerebrospinal, intraocular and synovial fluid)
♦ Fat.

Factors Affecting Distribution

Drugs can move between the compartments mainly through passive diffusion. The chemical nature of the drug will obviously be key in determining where it ends up, but there are several other factors that influence the rate and extent of this movement.

Perfusion of the compartment: As the drug is being carried in the blood, it is common sense that the amount of perfusion will influence how quickly a drug will distribute to a particular compartment. Drugs therefore tend to distribute most quickly in areas that are highly perfused. This includes the brain, the lungs and the heart. Over time, lipid-soluble drugs will redistribute to areas of fat that are normally poorly perfused.

Barriers between the compartments: The nature of the barrier separating the compartments is an important factor in terms of how easily the drugs move between these compartments. One important example of a barrier is the blood–brain barrier (see **Box 4.8**). This barrier is relatively impermeable, so presents a particular challenge to drug distribution.

Binding within the compartment: Drugs may become bound to proteins in a compartment, meaning that they are retained within that compartment. There is often extensive binding of the drug in the blood to plasma proteins, sometimes with less than 1% of the drug existing unbound and able to produce a pharmacological response. Changes in the levels of plasma protein and displacement of one drug by another can lead to changes in the levels of the unbound drug (see **Box 4.9**).

The relative hydrophilicity or lipophilicity of the drug: Drugs with a high lipid solubility, like morphine, are more likely to cross the blood–brain barrier. Other drugs, like gentamicin, have a low lipid solubility and therefore tend to stay in aqueous compartments.

Box 4.8 – Key information about the blood–brain barrier

♦ The function of the barrier is to protect the brain from damage by circulating chemicals.
♦ It consists of endothelial cells with tight junctions surrounded by pericytes.
♦ It is normally impermeable to many drugs and presents a challenge when formulating a medicine whose site of action is within the central nervous system (CNS).
♦ Small, lipid-soluble and unionised molecules pass through most readily.
♦ Inflammation can cause the barrier to become 'leaky' as its integrity is compromised. Drugs that would normally not have access can cross. Patients may be at risk of increased side effects.

Practice example:

♦ Methylnaltrexone is a μ-opioid receptor antagonist used for patients with opioid-induced constipation. It cannot cross the blood–brain barrier due to its low lipid solubility and polarity, and so only antagonises peripheral receptors located in the GI tract responsible for constipation. It cannot act on μ-opioid receptors in the brain so does not interfere with the analgesic effect of opioids.

Box 4.9 – Plasma protein binding

♦ Drugs can bind to binding sites on proteins that exist in the plasma.
♦ If the drug is bound to plasma proteins, then it is not free to interact with the drug target.
♦ Some drugs are extensively bound to proteins and so a large proportion of the dose taken may not reach the target.
♦ Usually this is not a problem, as any dose taken takes into account the normal level of protein binding.
♦ However, any reduction in the amount of plasma proteins in the body can lead to a higher than normal serum concentration of the drug.
♦ Clinically significant interactions due to displacement of the bound drug are most likely in drugs with a narrow therapeutic index (see below for more on the therapeutic index).
♦ Albumin is the most important plasma protein involved in binding drugs.

Volume of Distribution (Vd)

Vd can be confusing to understand initially as it refers to a theoretical volume rather than an actual volume per se. It is a concept used to describe the way in which drugs partition in the body by essentially comparing the way in which a drug actually distributes against its concentration in the plasma.

Definition:

The Vd is the volume of plasma that would be necessary to account for the total amount of a drug in the patient's body if that drug were present throughout the body at the same concentration as found in the plasma.

To illustrate this idea, we can compare two hypothetical drugs (see **Case Study 4.1**).

Metabolism

Following absorption and distribution, the body will begin to try to remove the drug from its system. The first step in this is metabolism, which is the chemical modification of the molecule usually in the liver. The reason that this is necessary is to make it easier for the body to eliminate. Often this means making the drug more water soluble as the primary route of elimination is via the kidneys.

In this section, we will focus on the two types of metabolic reaction, which often happen sequentially, and are called phase 1 and phase 2 reactions.

Case Study 4.1

The examples below are designed to illustrate what information can be gained from determining the Vd in terms of how drugs distribute in the body.

Drug A

500 micrograms of Drug A is given to a patient who weighs 70 kg. This drug is relatively water soluble and stays in the plasma. Levels show that peak plasma concentration is 30 mcg/L. In this patient, dividing the initial dose by the plasma concentration shows us that theoretically we would need 16.7 L to distribute the drug throughout the body at the same concentration. If we divide this by 70 kg, then we get a Vd of 0.24 L/kg.

Drug B

500 micrograms of Drug B is given to the same patient. This drug is relatively lipid soluble and distributes extensively outside the plasma. Levels show that peak plasma concentration is 1 mcg/L. Dividing the initial dose by plasma concentration shows that we would need 500 L of plasma to distribute the drug throughout the body at the same concentration. Dividing this by 70 kg, we get a Vd of 7.14 L/kg.

We can see that the amount of plasma needed to distribute Drug B is significantly greater than Drug A and so the Vd is much bigger. Whilst a large Vd does not tell us exactly where the drug distributes to, we know that it partitions into tissues or fluids outside of the plasma.

Phase 1 Reactions

These involve the chemical structure of the drug being altered through some kind of chemical reaction, such as oxidation, reduction or hydrolysis. The metabolites that are produced from phase 1 reactions fall into three pharmacological categories:

♦ A metabolite that has no pharmacological activity of its own is produced.
♦ A metabolite that retains some pharmacological activity, but less than that of the parent drug, is produced.
♦ A metabolite that is actually more pharmacologically active than the drug itself is produced.

The metabolites produced from drugs can therefore have an important role in their own right in the therapeutic action of a medicine.

Prodrugs

These are drugs that fall into the third category above and actually need to undergo metabolism to become pharmacologically active (see Box 4.10).

It is therefore not the drug but the **metabolite** that acts on a receptor target to produce or inhibit a physiological response. This method of drug delivery is useful for a range of reasons, including helping target drugs to a specific site of action or minimising side effects.

Box 4.10 – Examples of prodrugs

♦ Codeine is a prodrug of morphine. The codeine is metabolised *in vivo* to morphine.
♦ Enalapril is activated by a phase 1 reaction to enalaprilat.
♦ Azathioprine is metabolised to the active metabolite mercaptopurine.

Think about:

♦ Any drugs you will be prescribing that are either prodrugs or have active metabolites.
♦ What impact could a change in the metabolic capacity of the body have on their therapeutic effects?

Phase 2 Reactions

In phase 2 reactions, the drug or phase 1 metabolite has a molecule attached to it that increases its water solubility, making it easier to excrete from the body. The name given to this attachment is conjugation. Unlike phase 1 metabolites, the products of phase 2 reactions do not usually display any pharmacological activity.

The CYP450 Enzyme System

Enzymes play an important role in catalysing drug metabolism. A particularly important group of hepatic enzymes are the family of CYP450 enzymes. Within this group, there are various subsets of enzymes, known as isoforms, that are responsible for metabolising different drugs.

For example, carbamazepine is metabolised mainly by the CYP450 isoform CYP450 3A4 into its primary metabolite carbamazepine-10, 11-epoxide.

Changes in the capacity of these enzyme systems can lead to clinically significant changes in drug concentrations. Drugs can act to increase or decrease the amount of CYP450 enzymes, leading to potential drug interactions (see Box 4.11 for details).

Box 4.11 – Potential drug interactions with CYP450 enzymes

The change is known as ...	And the result is ...	Example
Enzyme **induction**	**Increased** synthesis of enzymes by the liver	Carbamazepine, phenytoin, sulphonylureas, rifampicin
Enzyme **inhibition**	**Decreased** synthesis of enzymes by the liver	Sodium valproate, cimetidine, ciprofloxacin, metronidazole

Think about:

♦ The prescribing of drugs that induce or inhibit CYP450 enzymes.
♦ These can lead to significant drug interactions.
♦ Because induction/inhibition can take some time to occur, make sure this is considered, even if a patient presents some time after the initiation of therapy.

Make you sure you become familiar with any enzyme inducers/inhibitors within your scope of practice.

Elimination

Once the drug has been broken down into a new chemical form, elimination can take place. This final step on the medicine's journey involves the physical removal of a drug or its metabolites from the body.

This can happen via the following routes.

Routes of Elimination:
♦ Urine
♦ Faeces
♦ Sweat
♦ Expired air.

How a drug is eliminated depends predominantly on the relative lipophilicity or hydrophilicity of the metabolites. As already discussed, drugs are hepatically metabolised primarily to produce water-soluble metabolites of lipid-soluble drugs. This means that most drugs are able to be excreted renally. Some water-soluble metabolites may be excreted by sweat or breast milk, but the amounts are usually relatively small. It is important, however, to consider breast milk in breast-feeding mothers due to the effect that the drug contained in the milk can have on the baby.

Anything that is not freely water-soluble moves via the bile duct into the gut and is then eliminated from the body via the faecal route. A complication of this route is the enterohepatic shunt (also known as enterohepatic circulation), whereby the drug/metabolite excreted in the bile can be reabsorbed from the GI tract, which can prolong its duration of action.

The Kinetics of Elimination

Drugs can be eliminated at different rates, and understanding this can support clinical decision making on, for example, dosing regimens or wash-out periods between drugs.

First Order Kinetics

This is the most straightforward model to understand and is the one that most drugs follow. In this model, the rate of metabolism is predictable and proportional to the concentration of the drug present.

It can be defined using the plasma half-life ($T_{1/2}$), where:

$T_{1/2}$ = the time taken for the concentration of drug to decrease by 50%.

To illustrate this, we can take a hypothetical drug – Drug A.

Imagine a patient has been taking Drug A which has a $T_{1/2}$ of 10 hours. This means it will take ten hours for the concentration of this drug to be reduced by 50% from its peak values. We will therefore see the following pattern of decreasing concentration:

Amount of drug present at time zero = 100%
Amount of drug present at ten hours (one half-life) = 50%
Amount of drug present at 20 hours (two half-lives) = 25%
Amount of drug present at 30 hours (three half-lives) = 12.5%
Amount of drug present at 40 hours (four half-lives) = 6.25%
Amount of drug present at 50 hours (five half-lives) = 3.125%

The amount remaining in the body will continue to decrease by 50% every ten hours until there is no drug left in the body. Usually it is considered that it will take approximately five half-lives for a drug to be reduced sufficiently for it to be removed from the body in terms of having any clinical relevance. This makes sense when we consider the information above that shows almost 97% of drug has been removed after five half-lives.

Example: The $T_{1/2}$ of amiodarone is approximately 50 days, although this varies considerably between patients. A $T_{1/2}$ of 100 days has been reported.

This means that five half-lives can be anywhere between 250 and 500 days. This information is important as it explains why there is therefore a risk that interactions with other drugs can occur long after treatment has ceased.

Zero Order Kinetics

A small number of drugs follow unpredictable metabolic kinetics, also known as saturation kinetics. This is because they involve metabolism by enzyme systems that can become saturated.

In the liver there are only a finite number of enzymes available to metabolise drugs that undergo zero order kinetics. This means that when you first start administering the drug, the enzymes will start filling up but there will be plenty spare. You can therefore keep increasing the amount of drug with the rate of metabolism staying constant. However, there comes a point where all the enzymes are occupied and the system becomes saturated. The rate of metabolism is limited because of the rate limiting step of the number of enzymes. At this point, a small increase in dose can lead to a large increase in drug concentrations. This of course is a problem when prescribing, as patients can have a small change in the dose prescribed, but if this tips them to the point where their enzymes are saturated, the resulting blood level can increase significantly. As patients can have varying amounts of metabolic enzymes, this can make the point of saturation difficult to predict.

Phenytoin is an example of a drug that undergoes zero order elimination, meaning that a small increase in dose can lead to a significant increase in serum concentration with the potential for drug toxicity.

Dose Response and Steady State

In this final section, we will look at the relationship between the administration of a dose and the response that is produced.

Dose Response

Figure 4.12 features a graph showing examples of what are known as dose response curves. These curves represent the typical relationship between the dose administered and the response that is produced. This shows response as a percentage of the maximum response against increasing dose. By plotting these graphs, we can compare the E_{max} and the ED_{50} of different drugs that produce similar effects. Figure 4.12 also demonstrates how we can use this to plot how types of drugs can affect response – in this instance, how a competitive antagonist affects the dose response of an agonist.

Reminder of what E_{max} and ED_{50} represent:

E_{max}: The dose that produces the maximal response of a drug
ED_{50}: The dose that produces 50% of the maximal response of a drug

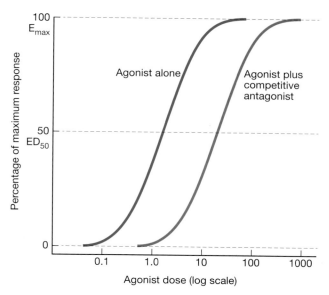

Figure 4.12 – Dose response curve

The response seen with an agonist makes sense when we think of it in the context of a biological system where response relies on drug–receptor interactions. Essentially what the curves show is that at very low doses there is a smaller effect on response. This is because the receptor binding sites are not occupied and only when a sufficient portion of them have been filled is a response seen. Once a sufficient number of binding sites are occupied, then the relationship between dose and response becomes essentially linear, as seen in the middle portion of the curve. At higher doses, the increase in response slows again as binding sites become increasingly filled and it is harder at this point for the agonist to find a vacant receptor site to bind to.

When a competitive antagonist is added to the system, we see a shift in the agonist dose response curve to the right. The maximal response that can be produced (E_{max}) does not change, but a higher dose is required to produce that response. The reason for this is that the effect of competitive antagonists can be overcome.

Example: To understand the relevance of this in practice, it may help to think about what impact this can have in the body.

Imagine there is an agonist that is actually an endogenous product – let's say a hormone – and there is a certain amount circulating in the body. If we imagine that the amount in circulation leads to a response that is equivalent to the ED_{50}, then under normal circumstances 50% of the maximal response will be produced. If we then administer a drug that is a competitive antagonist of this hormone, then it will mean that the circulating dose of hormone will no longer be able to produce 50% of the maximal response. However, if the body then increased production of this hormone to compensate, it would compete with the antagonist and the response could again reach the ED_{50}.

The addition of a competitive antagonist is only one example of how dose response can change, which should make sense when we think of the different types of drug receptor interactions there can be.

Antagonist alone: Antagonists have no efficacy, as they block the actions of agonists. If you plot a dose response curve of the antagonist alone, it will therefore be flat as no matter how much you increase the dose, no response will be seen (refer back to **Figure 4.3** for an illustration of this).

Partial agonists: These drugs produce a maximal response that is less than the maximal response produced by a full agonist. This means that the E_{max} and ED_{50} will both be less (refer back to **Figure 4.3** for an illustration of this).

Inverse agonist: As these produce a negative effect, the dose response curve becomes inverted into negative values.

A full discussion of all the ways in which dose response can be altered by various agonists/antagonists is beyond the scope of this book; for more on this, please see one of the pharmacology textbooks listed in the References and Further Reading section.

Steady State

It is important to remember that *in vivo* the drug is interacting with a whole range of processes and is normally given as repeated doses. This leads to a balance between the amount being administered and the amount being excreted. **Figure 4.13** shows a graph that illustrates what happens with repeated administration.

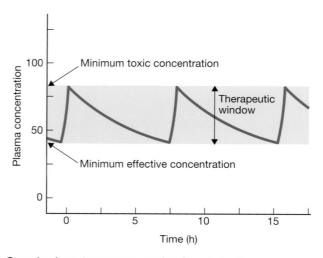

Figure 4.13 – Graph showing repeated administration

What this shows is that, with repeated dosing, there are fluctuations in plasma concentration over time; these are known as the peak and trough plasma concentrations. These are linked to factors such as how rapidly the dose is absorbed and distributed, metabolised and excreted. Despite these inevitable fluctuations, the peaks and troughs are consistent, meaning that on average the plasma concentration is at a level known as steady state.

Steady state is reached when the rate of absorption equals the rate of elimination.

It is important to appreciate that when a drug is initiated, serum levels do not immediately reach steady state. Thinking back to how drugs work, this is not surprising. Because metabolism and elimination occur following administration, several doses are usually needed to build up the concentrations at the receptor sites to produce the therapeutic levels needed.

Steady state is therefore usually reached after approximately three to five half-lives.

For example:

♦ Drug A has a half-life of five hours, so steady state will be reached after approximately 15–25 hours.
♦ Drug B has a half-life of 20 hours, so steady state will be reached after approximately 60–100 hours.

As well as steady state, **Figure 4.13** also highlights another pharmacological key term: therapeutic window (or therapeutic index). This term defines the range of serum concentrations at which a therapeutic response is seen. It is discussed further in the next section on therapeutic drug monitoring.

Key Points:
♦ The aim of treatment is to produce a therapeutic response, and normally there is a range of serum concentrations that will produce such a response.
♦ The minimum effective concentration is at the lower end of this range and any concentration below this is said to be subtherapeutic.
♦ Above the top end of this range, the dose becomes toxic.
♦ The range in the middle where the concentration is therapeutic is called the therapeutic index or window.

Loading Doses
If a fast response is needed, then a loading dose can be used to bring the serum concentration to within the therapeutic levels after a single dose. Subsequent doses will then keep the drug at steady state. These doses may be calculated individually for patients or more commonly a standard loading dose will be given.

Examples:

Digoxin given orally as a loading dose in atrial fibrillation or flutter is prescribed as a single dose of 0.75–1.5 milligrams. If there is an increased risk of adverse effects (e.g. in the elderly) or reduced urgency in treatment, then the dose can be divided and given six hours apart (see the SPC for digoxin and the BNF for further information).

Teicoplanin is a glycopeptide antibiotic used in gram-positive infections. It is administered either intravenously or intramuscularly. Loading doses are given to bring serum levels into therapeutic range. The first three doses are therefore loading doses and are given 12 hours apart. Further doses are then given every 24 hours (unless the patient has renal impairment when the dose interval may be extended).

Therapeutic Drug Monitoring (TDM)

Figure 4.14 highlights the concept that in practice ideally we want to prescribe drugs where the therapeutic window is wide and the peak effects are well below the top end of the therapeutic window. What this means is that the range of concentrations that produce a therapeutic effect is wide enough to allow a wide safety margin when doses are given between both toxic and subtherapeutic concentrations. The reason for this is because individuals process drugs in different ways and so the same dose of a drug given to different people may well not lead to equivalent serum concentrations. If the range of therapeutic concentrations is narrow, then there is a real risk of problems occurring in patients.

Most drugs have a relatively broad therapeutic window and so changes in serum concentration do not have a clinically significant impact (see Figure 4.14). There are some drugs that have a narrow therapeutic window, meaning that relatively small changes in serum concentration can have a clinical impact. This may be a loss of therapeutic control on the one hand or toxicity on the

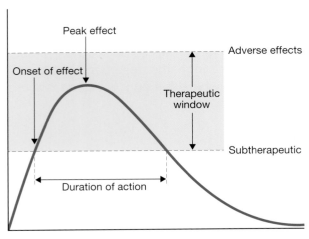

Figure 4.14 – Graph illustrating the therapeutic window

other. These drugs are used because they are so effective for the conditions for which they are prescribed. However, the risk to patients is minimised for this group of drugs by monitoring serum levels. Most NHS Trusts and Clinical Commissioning Groups (CCGs) will have policies and guidelines on TDM – make sure you know where to access your local guidance.

Examples of drugs with a narrow therapeutic index are:

♦ Phenytoin
♦ Gentamicin
♦ Carbamazepine
♦ Digoxin
♦ Lithium
♦ Vancomycin
♦ Theophylline
♦ Ciclosporin.

Think about:

Drugs with a narrow therapeutic window are high risk. You must always use caution when prescribing to someone on one of these medicines. You might not be prescribing the drug itself, but new medicines you prescribe may lead to changes in serum concentrations. If in doubt, seek advice.

Key Points:

♦ Time is taken for drug levels to reach steady state after repeated administration.
♦ Different doses will lead to different steady state levels, which may or may not be within the therapeutic window.
♦ For drugs that undergo zero order elimination at higher doses, steady state is not reached as there can be no equilibrium between absorption/elimination as the elimination system is saturated.

Conclusion

In this chapter, we have covered a range of concepts that you can use to help interpret information about the drugs you will be prescribing. Further reading is given below, with references to specific pharmacology textbooks which will give more detail on what has been covered. There are also links to websites which provide more information on drugs in practice. It is through exploring these resources, along with the local and national guidance, that you can build up your pharmacological knowledge and experience of the drugs that you will be working with. It may be useful to compile a personal formulary of drugs that you will be encountering, noting the key pharmacological aspects of these drugs.

Key Points of This Chapter

♦ Pharmacology is essential in understanding the mechanism of how drugs work and interact with the body.

♦ The concepts in this chapter can be applied to drugs you encounter in practice to enable you to be a safe and effective prescriber, though it will take time to build up knowledge and experience in your area of practice.

♦ Drugs act on targets in the body to produce some kind of physiological change.

♦ We can broadly group drugs into agonists and antagonists.

♦ Remember pharmacokinetic parameters using ADME — absorption, distribution, metabolism and elimination.

♦ Be cautious when changing therapy in patients when parameters such as bioavailability, therapeutic index or CYP450 metabolism may be affected.

References and Further Reading

Aulton, M. E. and Taylor, K. (2013) *Aulton's Pharmaceutics: The Design and Manufacture of Medicines*. Edinburgh: Churchill Livingstone.

Batchelder, A., Rodrigues, C. and Alrifari, A. (2011) *Rapid Clinical Pharmacolgy: A Student Formulary*. Chichester: Wiley-Blackwell.

Burton, M. E., Shaw, L. M., Schentag, J. J. et al. (2006) *Applied Pharmacokinetics and Pharmacodynamics: Principles of Therapeutic Drug Monitoring*. Baltimore, MD: Lippincott Williams & Wilkins.

Florence, A. and Attwood, D. (2011) *Physiochemical Principles of Pharmacy*. London: The Royal Pharmaceutical Society.

Gard, P. (2001) *Human Pharmacology*. London: CRC Press.

Katzung, B., Masters, S. and Trevor, A. (eds) (2012) *Basic and Clinical Pharmacology*. Maidenhead: McGraw-Hill.

Kenakin, T. P. (2017) *Pharmacology in Drug Discovery and Development: Understanding Drug Response*. Oxford: Elsevier/Academic Press.

Koup, J. (1989) Disease states and drug pharmacokinetics. *Journal of Clinical Pharmacology* 29: 674–679.

Li, J. et al. (2002) The Molecule Pages database. *Nature* 420: 716–717.

McFadden, R. (2009) *Introducing Pharmacology for Nursing and Healthcare*. Abingdon: Routledge.

Rang, H. P., Ritter, J.M., Flower, R. J. et al. (2016) *Rang & Dale's Pharmacology*. Oxford: Elsevier/Churchill Livingstone.

Rosenbaum, D. M., Rasmussen, S. G. F. and Kobilka, B. K. (2009) The structure and function of G-protein-coupled receptors. *Nature* 459(7245): 356–363.

Walker R. and Whittlesea, C. (eds) (2012) *Clinical Pharmacy and Therapeutics.* Oxford: Elsevier/Churchill Livingstone. (In particular, Chapter 3 entitled practical pharmacokinetics).

Useful Websites

The British National Formulary. This is the go-to reference for individual medicines and will give you brief information on anything important linked to prescribing that medicine. Available at: https://bnf.nice.org.uk.

The Electronic Medicines Compendium (eMC) is a database of the SPCs for medicines that are licensed in the UK. The SPC contains more detailed information than the BNF entries and is useful to refer to for learning and when you have a more complex patient. It has specific sections that cover the pharmacological properties of licensed medicines. Available at: https://www.medicines.org.uk/emc.

The National Institute for Clinical Excellence (NICE) includes guidance on various topics, such as managing ADRs and prescribing in renal disease. It is important to be aware of what guidance it has that may influence your practice, as it is a national NHS body producing evidence-based guidance. Available at: https://www.nice.org.uk.

NHS Specialist Pharmacy Services (SPS) is a website that has useful information on prescribing for staff working in the NHS. There are various articles that review evidence and aim to help prescribing decisions, particularly where there is limited evidence. Available at: https://www.sps.nhs.uk.

The online version of the Merck Manuals has a section on clinical pharmacology that you may find useful for general background info on pharmacological concepts. Available at: https://www.msdmanuals.com/professional/clinical-pharmacology.

Chapter 5
Prescribing in Special Groups

Jennifer Gorman

In This Chapter

- Introduction
- Renal impairment
- Liver impairment
- The elderly
- Patients with co-morbidities
- Palliative care patients
- Drug interactions
- Adverse drug reactions (ADRs)
- Individual Patient Variation: Pharmacogenetics
- Conclusion
- Key points of this chapter
- References and further reading
- Useful websites.

Introduction

Chapter 4 looked at the basics of pharmacology and what happens in general terms to drugs in the body. However, in practice, there are often variations in terms of how patients handle drugs pharmacologically and so treatment considerations vary in different patient groups. Depending on your scope of practice, some of these patient groups will be more or less relevant, but each section will discuss different pharmacological terms and should help consolidate your overall understanding of pharmacology. There is also a consideration of how patients' needs may differ between groups and some of the practical considerations there may be for you when prescribing.

The information provided is intended to give an overview of each area in order to provide an awareness of the general issues. If you will be prescribing in any of the specific groups discussed in this chapter, then you will need to ensure that you have the adequate level of education and competence before prescribing. This will of course include the practice-based aspect of your independent prescribing course, but references to further reading and resources are included to support your learning.

Renal Impairment

Chapter 4 highlighted how the elimination of drugs occurs mainly via the kidneys, meaning that renal impairment can have a significant impact on the pharmacokinetics of many drugs.

There are several ways in which renal impairment can cause problems for patients:

- **Drug toxicity:** If renal excretion of a drug or its metabolites is reduced, accumulation can occur. If serum levels are raised above the therapeutic window then toxicity can occur, leading to the patient suffering toxic effects. (For more on the therapeutic window, see **Chapter 4**.)
- **Increased sensitivity to some drugs:** This can mean that at standard doses patients may experience more ADRs.
- **Side effects may be more poorly tolerated:** Due to the effects of renal impairment, it may be that side effects have a greater clinical impact.
- **There can be a reduced level of efficacy:** It is obvious that there is a risk of toxicity from drugs that are renally cleared. However, if the drug requires concentrating within the urinary tract, then a reduced level of glomerular filtration may lead to reduced levels of drug at the site of action. This can cause reduced efficacy. An example of this is nitrofurantoin when used to treat urinary tract infections (UTIs).

How Do We Measure Renal Function?

Renal function calculations allow us to measure how well the kidneys are functioning in their ability to filter waste products from the blood. The design of the kidneys means that blood flows into the kidneys and through the glomeruli. It is in the glomeruli that glomerular filtration takes place and it is this process that forms the basis of the common measurements of renal function in practice. Figure 5.1 gives a reminder of the basic physiology of the kidney, showing the apparatus involved in glomerular filtration. If you need more of a reminder of how the kidneys work, then have a look at an anatomy and physiology book listed in the references.

Why Do We Use Creatinine?

There are various measures that can be used to calculate renal function, but the ones used commonly in practice have one thing in common: they use the endogenous product creatinine. Creatinine is actually nothing to do with renal function as such; it is a by-product of muscle breakdown. It is used as a way of evaluating the rate of glomerular filtration because usually the rate of muscle turnover is consistent. This means that if muscle turnover is stable, any change in the rate at which creatinine is filtered is usually due to a change in function

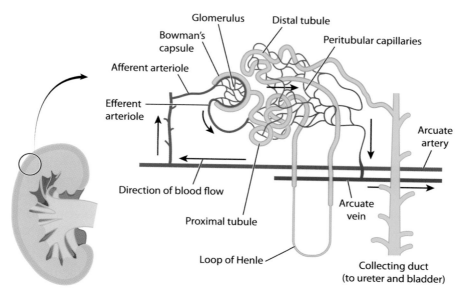

Figure 5.1 – Illustration of the nephrons of the kidney and renal blood supply, which are involved in the filtration and elimination of drugs
Source: © hfsimaging / 123RF.

of the kidney rather than the production of creatinine, if factors such as age and gender are taken into account. There are some exceptions to this rule, which are discussed later in the chapter.

The main measurement that is reported by laboratories, which you will likely already be familiar with, is the estimated glomerular filtration rate (eGFR). Many sources, such as the BNF, use eGFR when giving recommendations about adjusting drug therapy in renal impairment. This figure is estimated and is normalised to a body surface area of 1.73m². This means that in some patients an overestimation or underestimation of the glomerular filtration rate (GFR) may be seen with the eGFR.

Another way of calculating renal function is creatinine clearance (CrCl), using the Cockcroft and Gault equation. As can be seen from the formula below, age, weight and sex feature in this calculation.

The Cockcroft and Gault equation:

$$\text{Creatinine clearance ml/min} = \frac{(140 - \text{age}) \times \text{weight} \times \text{constant}}{\text{Serum Creatinine}}$$

♦ Age is in years
♦ Weight is in kilograms. Ideal body weight should be used where body fat is likely to be the main contributor to body mass
♦ Constant is dependent on sex, and = 1.23 for men and 1.04 for women
♦ Serum creatinine is in micromol/litre

Because of the different parameters used in these calculations, you must make sure that you use the right figure, as eGFR and CrCl are not interchangeable.

Factors That Can Affect the Reliability of Renal Function Calculations

Overall, there is not one measure that is superior to another in all patient populations or clinical situations. In certain patient groups, CrCl is the preferred measure, as it gives a higher degree of accuracy; see below for more information. In the majority of the population who are within average ranges of muscle mass, eGFR gives a reliable estimate of renal function. The reason for this is that the estimated figures used in eGFR calculations are based on average population characteristics. As the elimination of creatinine can change in certain circumstances, estimations based on average characteristics are not always reliable.

The BNF (2019) also lists the following as times when you should use caution or not use creatinine as a measure of renal function at all:

♦ As serum creatinine is dependent on muscle mass, measurements should be interpreted with caution in those who have levels of muscle mass that deviate from the norm, e.g. the elderly, bodybuilders or amputees.
♦ Acute illness that leads to rapid changes in renal function means that creatinine is not a useful measure of renal function.
♦ Creatinine is also not a useful proxy for renal function in patients with acute kidney injury (AKI).

Think about:

How you can improve safe prescribing in patients who have or are at risk of developing renal impairment:

♦ **Nephrotoxic drugs:** Always be cautious about using drugs that can be nephrotoxic in patients with pre-existing renal impairment due to the risk of serious consequences.
♦ **Patients who are acutely unwell:** NICE advises that during intercurrent illness, the risk of acute kidney injury is increased in patients with an eGFR of less than 60 ml/min/1.73 m^2. Potentially nephrotoxic or renally excreted drugs may require dose reduction or temporary discontinuation.
♦ **Drugs with a narrow therapeutic index:** These require special care in renal impairment – make sure you are familiar with these drugs and, if necessary, get advice when prescribing for a patient on one of these.
♦ **Where you will look for information and advice when you become a prescriber:** e.g. the SPC, the BNF, *The Renal Drug Handbook* and other team members – depending on where you work, this may include more experienced colleagues, pharmacists or perhaps the renal team.

It is recommended that CrCl is used to measure renal function in all patients over 75 years old because of age-related physiological changes, which will be discussed later in this chapter. It is also the preferred method in patients at extremes of muscle mass.

For a more detailed discussion of estimating renal function, please see the references and further reading section, e.g. the 'prescribing in renal impairment' section in the BNF (2019) or UKMi Medicines Q&A 167.6 (NHS UKMi, 2016).

Dosing in Renal Impairment

Measurement of renal function can be used to inform dose adjustments. There are different ways that dosing regimens can be altered to avoid toxicity if drug accumulation is a risk:

♦ Standard dose given at extended intervals
♦ Reduced dose given at the usual intervals
♦ A combination of dose reduction and extended interval.

Box 5.1 provides some examples.

Information on the best way to manage changes in dosing can be found in a variety of sources, such as the SPC and the BNF. *The Renal Drug Handbook* is an invaluable source of information for managing prescribing for patients with renal impairment. It contains monographs for individual drugs, giving detailed pharmacological information and practical advice on dose adjustments (see the references and further reading section at the end of the chapter for full details of this title).

Box 5.1 – Examples of altering dosing regimens in renal impairment

♦ Teicoplanin is an antibiotic given parenterally for gram-positive infections, such as cellulitis. In renal impairment it is the dose interval of maintenance treatment that is changed rather than the dose itself.
♦ Ramipril is recommended to be started at the lowest dose of 1.25 milligrams, given once daily as usual. The dose is then titrated according to the response.

Case Study 5.1

You are visiting Mr Patel, a 72-year-old patient in his home. He has an infected wound on his left arm that requires dressing. He mentions that he is suffering from pain and is wondering if there is anything he can take.

PMH: type 2 diabetes, mild asthma

Drug history: metformin 500 milligrams TDS, salbutamol 100 micrograms MDI 2 puffs PRN

You take a history and conduct an examination. You find that the pain is linked to swelling and inflammation around the infected area on the patient's arm as well as some muscle pain associated with the fall that caused the wound. The patient has been initiated on flucloxacillin 500 milligrams QDS (as per local guidelines), and the patient has only taken two doses so far. You conclude that there are no red flags and analgesia can be used to manage the pain.

Question: What other information would you want to know before prescribing for the patient?

Answer: Allergy status. Whether any OTC medicines/herbal remedies are being taken. Also, because of the patient's age and the fact that he is diabetic and thus prone to renal impairment, when the last U&Es were taken and what they were.

Question: You find after checking the clinical system that the patient has mild renal impairment (eGFR = 55 ml/min/1.73 m^2). Would this change your prescribing, and if so how?

Answer: Usually simple analgesia such as paracetamol and an NSAID would be prescribed. However, NSAIDs can cause AKI and this patient is diabetic and already has renal impairment with an eGFR of 55 ml/min/1.73 m^2. He is also at risk because if he does develop AKI, then there is the possibility that the metformin he is prescribed could cause lactic acidosis if his eGFR goes below 45 ml/min/1.73 m^2. There is also the unrelated issue that NSAIDs can cause bronchospasm and this patient is asthmatic. It is only an issue in approx. 10% of patients and often patients have taken them OTC without any problem – however, it would need checking.

In this case it is likely that the risk of prescribing outweighs the benefit and prescribing paracetamol alongside non-pharmacological therapy is indicated. Low-dose codeine is a possibility if paracetamol alone does not control the pain, but you need to be mindful of the risk of falls in the elderly as well as the potential for constipation. It is important to consider any local prescribing guidelines.

Liver Impairment

The liver is a complex organ that is responsible for a range of homeostatic functions within the human body. This means that liver impairment can have an important impact on the pharmacology of drugs. For example, the liver is involved in synthesising proteins, such as plasma proteins and clotting factors. Albumin is a plasma protein produced in the liver, which is important in the context of protein binding of drugs within the plasma. The liver also plays an important role in the metabolism of drugs through phase 1 and phase 2 metabolic reactions (see **Chapter 4**). Some of the other main impacts of liver impairment on drug handling in the body are summarised in Table 5.1. The clinical impact of each of these different factors is of course dependent on both the type and severity of the liver disease.

Table 5.1 – Some of the key problems of prescribing in patients with liver disease

Problem	Consequence
Reduction in hepatic metabolism	Impaired metabolism can lead to accumulation and to drug toxicity.
Hypoproteinaemia	Decreased synthesis of plasma proteins and subsequent hypoproteinaemia can lead to changes in distribution of highly protein-bound drugs.
Changes in drug distribution due to fluid overload (e.g. with oedema or ascites)	Water-soluble drugs can potentially distribute into oedematous and ascitic fluid. This may cause a reduction in drug concentration at the site of action. This can be exacerbated when drugs that cause fluid retention are prescribed.
Lack of activation of prodrugs	Prodrugs requiring activation in the liver may have a reduced therapeutic effect due to a decrease in the rate or extent of activation. If the activated drug is metabolised in the liver this can, however, lead to reduced elimination. So, essentially there may be less active drug circulating, but it may be eliminated more slowly than usual. This means the clinical effect can be unpredictable.
Changes in the first pass metabolism of drugs	This can lead to altered bioavailability of medications. If a drug is usually highly metabolised by the first pass effect, then the bioavailability can be increased in liver impairment.
Drugs precipitating hepatic encephalopathy	In severe disease, drugs can affect cerebral function which can precipitate hepatic encephalopathy.
Hepatotoxicity	Patients with pre-existing liver disease may be more prone to both dose-related and idiosyncratic hepatotoxicity caused by certain drugs.

(*continued*)

Table 5.1 – Some of the key problems of prescribing in patients with liver disease (*continued*)

Problem	Consequence
Changes in drug elimination	Drugs that are excreted in the bile may have reduced excretion in cholestatic patients. Enterohepatic circulation of drugs can also be affected.
Reduction in the synthesis of clotting factors by the liver	A raised INR (Internationalised Normalised Ratio) is an indicator of impaired metabolic capacity and is seen in severe impairment. There will also be increased sensitivity to any drugs that affect clotting. Patients will need specialist input to ensure prescribing is appropriate.

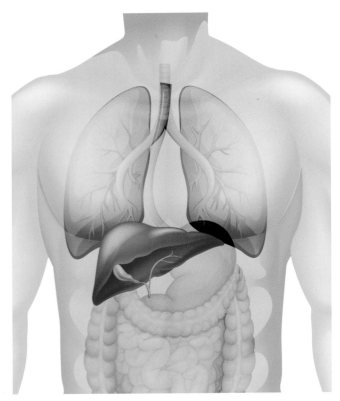

Figure 5.2 – Prescribing in hepatic impairment can change a patient's handling of drugs in complex ways
Source: © bluering media / 123RF.

Assessing Liver Function

The liver has a large reserve capacity, meaning that it is unlikely that clinically significant changes in drug action will be seen unless the impairment is severe. A complication of using liver function tests (LFTs) to adjust drug therapy is that routine LFTs are not reliable as predictors of which drugs may display impaired metabolism. There is also variation between patients. As the liver has such varied functions and the causes of liver impairment can vary considerably, any changes can be complex and multifactorial.

The other challenge is the lack of an endogenous marker equivalent to creatinine with which the effect of liver dysfunction on excretion can be quantified. This means that making decisions about dose adjustment is more complex than in renal impairment. There are a range of LFTs that give different pieces of the picture of the liver's function. All these factors combine to make it incredibly hard to make generalisations about prescribing at appropriate doses in patients with this condition.

Because of this, in all patients with severe disease, prescribing should be kept to a minimum.

The BNF (see **Box 5.2**) features general guidance on prescribing in hepatic impairment, as well as information on individual drugs.

A thorough review of the pharmacodynamic and pharmacokinetic implications on prescribing produced by UKMi is available from the Specialist Pharmacy Service (2014). It is not advocated that you would be making decisions on whether to prescribe at this level of complexity. However, it may be useful to help consolidate your pharmacology knowledge as it is a good example of how pharmacological principles can be applied in prescribing practice.

Drugs as a Cause of Liver Impairment

It is important to remember that, as a prescriber, some of the drugs you will prescribe can themselves potentially cause liver problems. In fact, an important cause of liver impairment is the prescribing of drugs, with approximately 20–30% of acute liver failure linked to drug use (Walker and Whittlesea 2018).

Box 5.2 – Example of information on prescribing in hepatic impairment from the BNF

Warfarin: 'Avoid in severe impairment, especially if prothrombin time is already prolonged.'

See: https://bnf.nice.org.uk/drug/warfarin-sodium.html#hepaticImpairment

---

Drugs that can cause liver damage are known as hepatotoxic. The damage can either be dose-related or idiosyncratic, which means it is unrelated to the dose. The types of problems that can occur vary widely, including acute hepatitis, fatty liver and cholestasis. It is clear that hepatotoxic drugs should not be prescribed in patients with known liver disease unless under specialist guidance. However, the situation is more complex when prescribing for patients without liver disease and the risk of the drug causing liver impairment should be weighed against the clinical risk. For example, if an otherwise fit and well person needs an antibiotic for a severe infection and the antibiotic has a low risk of causing liver impairment then the benefit would certainly seem to outweigh the risk. However, if a patient has multi-morbidity and is on multiple medicines already, then prescribing an additional medicine that has a high risk of hepatotoxicity would require more thought.

If a medicine is initiated, then appropriate monitoring should be done of LFTs to ensure any adverse effects on the liver are detected. For example, routine LFTs are required every 2 to 3 months for patients stabilised on methotrexate when used at low doses for inflammatory diseases like rheumatoid arthritis (RA).

Think about:

Why are changes in serum concentration that are due to changes in protein synthesis and subsequent protein binding in hepatic impairment particularly significant for phenytoin?

Answer: Because it has a narrow therapeutic index and undergoes zero order elimination. This means that relatively small increases in free drug can lead to large increases in serum concentration and thus toxicity.

The Elderly

Changes in the functioning of the body occur throughout life and as the human body ages, it demonstrates complex changes that can impact on the pharmacological handling of medicines. It is important to understand that ageing is not uniform or consistent. It represents the sum of a variety of changes that occur at different rates in different individuals. It involves functional decline as well as a variety of anatomical and physiological changes, all of which can lead to changes in the pharmacological response of an individual.

An important factor in the older population is the increased propensity for co-morbidities and polypharmacy (for more on co-morbidities, see later in this chapter; for more on polypharmacy, see **Chapter 11** on medicines optimisation). This is in addition to the changes that happen as a natural part of ageing. Figure 5.3 illustrates that functional decline generally begins in the forties and continues in a roughly linear trajectory into old age. It is important to

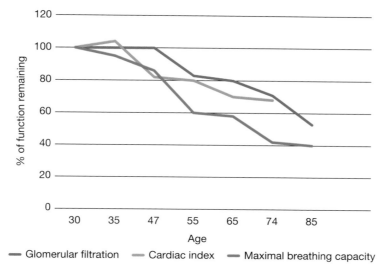

Figure 5.3 – The effect of age on some physiological functions
Source: Based on data from Katzung et al. (2012).

Table 5.2 – Some age-related changes in pharmacokinetics

Variable	Young adults (20–30 years)	Older adults (60–80 years)
Body water (% of body weight)	61	53
Lean body mass (% of body weight)	19	12
Body fat (% of body weight)	26–33 (women) 18–20 (men)	38–45 (women) 36–38 (men)
Serum albumin (g/dL)	4.7	3.8
Kidney weight (% of young adult)	(100)	80
Hepatic blood flow (1% of young adult)	(100)	55–60

Source: Katzung et al. (2012, p. 1052).

remember that functional change is very variable and the data presented in **Figure 5.3** represents mean figures. **Table 5.2** shows some of the physiological and anatomical changes that can also occur, which affect the pharmacokinetic handling of drugs.

Pharmacokinetic Changes

The parameters shown in **Table 5.2** make it clear how pharmacokinetic parameters can be altered by these age-related changes.

The proportion of body fat and water changes considerably with age: the proportion of fat increases and the proportion of water decreases. As discussed in **Chapter 4**, the distribution of a drug depends on whether it is lipophilic or hydrophilic. Such changes in body composition can then lead to a change in drug distribution.

Another parameter that can affect distribution is serum albumin. A reduction in the synthesis of albumin levels can cause serum levels of drugs that are highly protein-bound to increase. This is usually only clinically significant in drugs that have a narrow therapeutic index.

Blood flow to the liver in elderly patients is reduced to approximately 55–60% of that of a young adult. As blood flow is a determinant in the hepatic clearance of drugs from the blood, it follows that the rate of the removal of a drug from the body may be reduced. As we have already discussed, however, the liver is a complex organ and it is difficult to quantify precisely what clinical impact these changes may have.

Kidney weight in adults aged 60–80 is on average only 80% that of a young adult. This is linked to loss of nephrons in the kidney and means that older people will usually have some degree of renal impairment. Patients over 80 years old can be assumed to have renal impairment due to this functional decline (Whittlesea and Walker 2018). As outlined in **Chapter 4**, the aim of metabolism is essentially to make drugs more water soluble, because renal clearance of drugs is the most common route of excretion. Age-related changes in renal impairment can have significant effects on renal clearance.

Pharmacodynamic Changes

Elderly patients appear to show increased sensitivity to the pharmacodynamic effects of certain drugs. In many instances it is unclear exactly why this is the case. It may be that it is due to pharmacokinetic processes that have not yet been elucidated. Whatever the reason, clinical studies do show that the elderly are more sensitive to many commonly used drugs.

Examples of drugs that elderly patients display increased sensitivity to include:

♦ Benzodiazepines
♦ Antipsychotics
♦ Antiparkinsonian drugs
♦ NSAIDs
♦ Antihypertensives.

Key Considerations When Prescribing to the Elderly

Because of the pharmacological differences seen in the elderly, extra care is needed when prescribing:

♦ Make sure you have the competence to know how the drugs you are prescribing affect elderly patients. The BNF suggests prescribers limit the range of medicines they prescribe in the elderly to ones with which they are thoroughly familiar.

♦ Consider whether pharmacological management is needed – is there a non-pharmacological option that would be appropriate? For example, diuretics used chronically are over-prescribed. They should not be prescribed for gravitational oedema for more than a few days. Instead, increased movement, elevation and support stockings should normally be used.

♦ Make sure appropriate follow-up and review is in place. Medicines should be monitored and reviewed regularly. Any medicines no longer deemed appropriate should be de-prescribed. For example, if NSAIDs are indicated short-term, make sure they are stopped as soon as possible due to the risk of AKI with this class of drugs.

♦ Consider using a tool to help support reviewing and stopping medicines, e.g. the STOPP/START tool (see **Chapter 11** for more on this).

♦ Consider the risk-benefit ratio when prescribing; this may change in elderly patients.

♦ Consider the patient as a whole, including co-morbidities, all medication currently taken and the degree of age-related change in that patient.

For further support on this topic, see the references given at the end of the chapter.

The section in the BNF on prescribing for the elderly contains a useful summary that is easy to refer to and includes more detail on the different measurements of renal function.

Patients with Co-morbidities

Prescribing in patients with co-morbidities can present a huge challenge, but from your previous experience you will know it is one that it is likely you will encounter frequently. When prescribing, you need to consider the drugs currently prescribed, the co-morbidities the patient has and then how the drug you wish to prescribe might affect these. You also need to consult the patient about their expectations of treatment outcomes and perceptions about the proposed medication.

There is no 'one size fits all' approach to prescribing in this group, as each patient can present with a different mixture of conditions and drugs. Guidelines and formularies that help support prescribing have limitations in this group, as often they will be focused on managing a condition in isolation. This means that targets set for treatment outcomes may not be suitable for patients with co-morbidities. Knowledge of the pharmacology of drugs can help, as by looking at the mechanism of action of a drug or its side effects you can make judgements on whether it is clinically appropriate in a specific patient.

The prescribing of multiple medicines in an individual patient is known as polypharmacy. In patients with co-morbidities, polypharmacy is, unsurprisingly, commonly seen. The term polypharmacy has certain negative connotations and certainly there are instances where multiple medicines are prescribed inappropriately. There is a risk that a prescribing cascade could happen, where a patient is prescribed a drug, this causes a side effect and so another drug is prescribed to counteract that. This cascade can then spiral out of control. However, polypharmacy can also be appropriate and in patients with co-morbidities, multiple medicines can often be needed to manage the patient's conditions effectively (Cahill 2015; Payne et al. 2014). The skill as a prescriber comes in being able to evaluate whether the polypharmacy in a particular patient is appropriate or inappropriate.

To do this, you need to be particularly clear about the rationale for prescribing, taking into account the fact that the risk and benefit of treatments may differ from patients presenting with single conditions. This means considering what you are trying to achieve with treatment and what outcome you are looking for. Using an approach that takes into account the patient's quality of life, preferences and values is therefore very important in this group of patients (Tinetti et al. 2004). It may mean, for example, changing the goal of treatment from reducing conventional disease markers to improving quality of life (Cahill 2015).

Turn to **Chapter 11** for more on polypharmacy and shared decision making

Palliative Care Patients

It is likely that in your role you will need to prescribe for patients who require ongoing palliative care and those who are entering the final phase of their life. Traditionally, district nurses have had a high level of input into this group of patients. It has been estimated that 'around 40% of a district nurse's work is devoted to caring for patients with palliative care needs' (Faull et al 2012). Becoming a prescriber, however, brings a new set of challenges in this specialist area. It is important to remember that whatever your role, this group of patients benefits from teamworking in the community setting (Faull et al. 2012). It is therefore useful to develop your links with both GPs and specialist teams in your local area.

Clinical Assessment of the Patient

Clinical assessment of palliative care patients requires a high level of skill. This is because the trajectory of disease progression in different conditions and in different patients can be very unpredictable. As prescribing decisions are influenced by weighing the benefits and risks of treatment, this uncertainty can make prescribing challenging. For example, if a patient has a chronic condition, determining whether you are treating an exacerbation of their condition or whether the patient is indeed entering the final stage of their disease can alter how you prescribe. NICE guideline NG31: Care of dying adults in the last days of life has a section entitled 'Recognising when a person may be in the last days of life' (NICE 2015). This provides recommendations that act to supplement your clinical judgement in helping you decide if a patient is at the end of their life.

Whatever your clinical assessment determines, you should make decisions about prescribing jointly with the patient and possibly family/carers if appropriate.

Drug Choice, Dose, Route and Formulation

The nature of prescribing in this group of patients means that therapy should be tailored to the needs of the patient. The purpose of treatment in the palliative patient is slightly different as it is predominantly to reduce symptoms and improve quality of life rather than improve clinical markers of disease or extend life. As each patient will present with a different set of symptoms and different expectations about their management, a patient-centred approach is essential. A detailed review of all the drugs used in this area of practice is beyond the scope of this text, but further reading is given at the end of the chapter for you to expand your knowledge. Local guidelines should always be referred to when prescribing.

A wide range of drugs is used for symptom management; some examples include analgesics, antiemetics and drugs for agitation and excessive respiratory secretions. See the BNF section on prescribing in palliative care for an overview of the types of symptoms and drugs used to manage them (BNF, 2020). The drugs prescribed can lead to a whole host of side effects, and the balance of managing symptoms with side effects needs to be discussed with the patient, family and/or carer. As these effects are often due to predictable pharmacological responses, such as sedation with opioids or constipation with anticholinergics, they can be dose-related. This means doses should be regularly reviewed and titrated as needed.

National and local clinical guidelines should be used to support the choice of drug prescribed, along with aspects such as dosing, titrating and monitoring treatment. NICE clinical guideline CG140 is an example of one such guideline as it focuses on the prescribing of strong opioids in palliative care. It provides basic advice on drug choice and titrating doses. Another common issue when prescribing is switching between drugs. It may be that you need to switch between opioid drugs as a patient's analgesia needs and physical condition change. The BNF section on prescribing in palliative care has a useful section on dose conversions. Other key references include the Palliative Care Formulary (Twycross et al. 2018) and of course any local formularies used in your area. Ensure you are confident in the drugs you are using before prescribing and if you are unsure, seek specialist advice.

Turn to **Chapter 6** for more general information on managing pain.

There are specific patient factors that may be altered due to the presence of terminal illness, which could mean dosing needs to be adjusted. Changes in body weight and composition may occur, for example in patients presenting with cachexia. Liver or renal impairment can also be present as a result of their condition or other co-morbidities. Access to recent bloods is therefore important when assessing patients' medication, but they may be difficult to obtain out of hours and you need to consider how to deal with this. Hospices may have phonelines that healthcare professionals can access out of hours for support, so it may be that you can access some information from the local hospice if the patient is already known to them.

The route and formulation of drugs will also need to be carefully considered to ensure they are suitable for the patient. Generally, the oral route is preferred over parenteral unless there is severe nausea and vomiting, dysphagia, weakness or coma. There is a wide range of drugs available that come in a range of oral formulations. Morphine, for example, comes as modified release tablets/capsules as well as immediate release tablets and liquid that can be used for breakthrough pain. This means dosing can easily be reviewed and optimised. Using an analgesic opioid patch, such as fentanyl, can be helpful for patients with gastric problems or swallowing difficulties. However, they are only suitable in patients that have stable pain and are not suitable for patients who have acutely changing analgesic requirements. It is also worth remembering that there are other non-parenteral routes that do not rely on absorption in the GI tract, such as buccal, sublingual and rectal. These may be useful for some patients.

For more on steady state serum concentrations, turn to **Chapter 4**.

Another consideration when prescribing in palliative care is that medicines are used more often outside of licence than in some other areas of practice. About 25% of prescribing in palliative care in the UK has in the past been found to be off-label (Atkinson and Kirkham 1999; Todd and Davies 1999). Drugs can be used for indications that they are not licensed for, such as some anti-epileptics used for neuropathic pain. Drug formulations can also be altered and used off label or may be given by an unlicensed route.

For example, if a patient is unable to tolerate oral feed, they may have a percutaneous endoscopic gastroscopy (PEG) inserted. The obvious choice in this situation may seem to switch everything to liquids, but this is not always the best option. Some liquids are actually more prone to block enteral tubes, and dispersible tablets may be better. Sometimes there may not be a licensed liquid that can be used anyway, so tablets might have to be crushed or even injections used enterally. Another consideration is that there can be interactions between drugs going into the tube and even between a drug and the plastic the tube is made from. Specialist information sources are available to support prescribing (Smyth 2015; White and Bradnam 2015). These are usually used by pharmacists and you should seek advice if prescribing in this area. This can be through a pharmacist or your local hospice, depending on your local arrangements. As well as the clinical aspects of off-label prescribing, you also need to consider the legal and ethical implications of this and the involvement of the patient in decisions.

Turn to **Chapter 9** for more on law and ethics.

Prescribing for Syringe Drivers

Syringe drivers can be a useful option in palliative care if patients become unable to tolerate medicines. It is a less painful option than repeated IM injections and it is easier and with less risk of infection compared with cannulating a patient to access the IV route. The SC continuous infusion administered by this method results in stable steady state serum concentrations of drugs that can provide good symptom control. Analgesics, sedatives, anticholinergics and antiemetics can all be given via this route. They can be prescribed individually or combined into one syringe driver. Combining multiple drugs does require knowledge about the compatibility of drugs. Some drugs can be used together but may only be compatible at certain concentrations, whilst some are not compatible at all. Palliative care specialist texts such as palliativedrugs.com and local guidelines can provide support with common combinations of drugs. It is always worth checking with a specialist locally if you are prescribing drugs that you have not prescribed together before, or if it is an unusual combination. It is also worth considering the possible alternatives to putting medicines in a syringe driver. For example, dexamethasone is a steroid and in common with other steroids can disturb sleep. Adding it to a continuous infusion may be detrimental to the patient, and because the drug has a long half-life (Dexamethasone 3.3 milligrams/ml SPC, available at: https://www.medicines. org.uk/emc/product/4659/smpc) it can be given by a bolus SC injection instead.

For more on the pros and cons of different formulations, turn to **Chapter 4**.

Practicalities of Prescribing in This Group of Patients

Providing best practice palliative care is not just about ensuring the most clinically appropriate medicines are prescribed, but also includes some more practical aspects of how the drugs are accessed by patients and administered.

One key issue faced by prescribers is access to medicines for their patients. Planning the quantity needed, particularly in the out-of-hours period, can be difficult, as doses can be hard to predict. There is a balance between ensuring the patient does not run out of drugs and needless wastage. It is useful to consider from a prescriber's perspective how your patients can access drugs when they need them. Many community pharmacies do not carry stocks of the drugs used routinely in palliative care as they can be too bulky to fit into controlled drug cabinets and may not commonly be dispensed. Pharmacies can usually get medicines either on the same day, or on the next day if they don't stock them, so the patient's usual pharmacy should be the first port of call for routine prescribing. It is, however, important to know where you can signpost your patients and their families/carers to access drugs in case of an emergency. In some areas, certain local pharmacies hold an agreed stock of drugs used in palliative care for emergency situations. As stocks are often limited, it is intended this is used for emergencies only and does not replace routine planned care. Other areas issue prepared boxes of medicines to be kept in the patients' homes that can be used 'just in case'. Ensure you find out what provision has been made in your local area.

It is worth noting the practical challenge that can be faced by district nurse prescribers where there may be an expectation that the district nurse will administer the drugs once they have been prescribed, due to time or staffing issues. This is something you need to discuss with your manager and ideally have a plan for in advance.

The final practical consideration is around the prescription itself and any prescription charts. These can be very complicated and often include controlled drugs. Any errors in the paperwork can involve time and delay in rectifying due to tight controlled drugs regulations, so ensure you take time to become very familiar with the legal requirements for these.

Developing your skills in this area of practice has the potential to support access to medicines for patients who need symptom management. The knowledge and experience that district nurses can bring to palliative care also have the potential to deliver holistic, patient-centred care and end-of-life best practice.

> ## Think about:
>
> ♦ How are you going to develop your knowledge and skills in prescribing for patients at the end of their life?
> ♦ Do you know what services there are locally to support you? If so, do you know how to access them both in and out of hours?
> ♦ How will your prescribing take into account the quantities needed to ensure the patient doesn't run out of medication, particularly in the out-of-hours period?

Drug Interactions

Because patients are often prescribed multiple medicines, it is important to be aware of the possibility of interactions and know how to manage them. Drug interactions happen when the effect of a drug is changed by the presence of another drug, a chemical or even food.

Pharmacodynamic Interactions

These interactions occur when drugs have either similar or antagonistic pharmacological effects. If, for example, two drugs are given that both cause sedation, then this can have an additive effect.

Clinical examples of this type of drug interaction:

♦ Atenolol and tamsulosin: These are used for different indications. Atenolol is a beta-blocker used for its cardiac effects. Tamsulosin is an alpha-blocker used for urinary retention. Both, however, can lower the blood pressure, potentially leading to hypotension.
♦ Diazepam and mirtazapine: Both have CNS depressive effects, which can have an additive effect producing CNS effects such as increased drowsiness.
♦ Warfarin and aspirin: This interaction increases the risk of bleeds due to an additive effect of anticoagulant and antiplatelet action of the drugs.

This type of interaction is normally predictable based on the known pharmacology of the drug.

Pharmacokinetic Interactions

These interactions occur when one drug alters the absorption, distribution, metabolism or elimination of another drug. Because of the complex nature of pharmacokinetic effects, it may not always be possible to easily predict these interactions. Common examples of this kind of interaction may be interactions caused by the induction or inhibition CYP450 enzyme systems that were discussed in **Chapter 4**.

Clinical examples of pharmacokinetic drug interactions:

♦ Bisphosphates and calcium supplements: Calcium is predicted to reduce absorption of bisphosphates and so a gap is recommended between ingestion of the different drugs.
♦ Simvastatin and grapefruit juice: Grapefruit juice increases levels of simvastatin due to changes in metabolic enzymes, leading to the possibility of severe side effects, including rhabdomyolysis.
♦ Doxycycline and iron supplements: Iron should be taken 2–3 hours after tetracycline antibiotics such as doxycycline, as it decreases the absorption of these antibiotics.

When you are faced with the possibility of having to prescribe two interacting drugs, it is important to consider the options, including the risk-benefit ratio of prescribing. Some factors to consider when there is the possibility of drug interactions are as follows:

♦ What information is there on how common the interaction is?
♦ How severe are the consequences of the interaction if it occurs?
♦ Is the interaction dose-related and can the risk be minimised by a dose reduction?
♦ Are there other drugs that do not interact that could achieve the same therapeutic outcome?
♦ If a short course of treatment is needed, can an interacting drug be temporarily stopped?
♦ Is there any monitoring that can be done to check for the development of an interaction?

Adverse Drug Reactions (ADRs)

The World Health Organization's definition of an ADR is a noxious, unintended or undesired effect of a drug when used at therapeutic doses (WHO, 1972). This means it does not include toxic reactions produced by above-therapeutic doses, which have been taken either intentionally or un-intentionally.

The definition was written in 1972 by the World Health Organization in a report produced in response to the growing problem of ADRs. Unfortunately, even with increased safety monitoring of drugs, ADRs continue to be of huge significance in practice. Box 5.3 below gives an idea of the burden of ADRs to both patients and the NHS. As a prescriber, it is your responsibility to try where possible to identify patients who may be at risk of an ADR and also to correctly manage patients who present with an ADR. As we will see, this is not always an easy task and so taking time to familiarise yourself with this topic is important.

What the information in Box 5.3 shows is the frequency of ADRs and the potential severity, but also highlights that many ADRs were in fact preventable based on knowledge of their pharmacology.

Box 5.3 – Summary of key findings from a study investigating the burden of ADRs on patients and the NHS

♦ ADRs account for 1 in 16 hospital admissions and 4% of NHS bed capacity.
♦ 70% of ADRs were considered to be avoidable.
♦ Many ADRs were predictable based on the pharmacology of the drugs involved and were therefore likely to be preventable.
♦ 1 in 6 ADRs was due to drug interactions.
♦ Admissions caused by ADRs led to mortality in 2% of patients.
♦ ADRs may be the cause of death in 0.15% of all patients admitted to hospital (this figure is consistent with data from the US).

Source: Pirmohamed et al. (2004).

Case Study 5.2

You go to see Mrs B, a 66-year-old patient who has a one-week history of purulent cough.

PMH: hypercholesteremia, hypertension

Drug history: amlodipine 10 milligrams once daily, simvastatin 20 milligrams every night

Allergies: penicillin

Following a full history and physical examination, you diagnose that he has a low-severity community-acquired pneumonia.

Question: Based on the NICE guidelines for diagnosing and managing pneumonia, what treatment will you recommend?

Answer: Ideally, treatment should be with a penicillin, such as amoxicillin, for five days. In penicillin-allergic patients, a macrolide should be used. In penicillin allergic patients either clarithromycin or doxycycline can be used.

Question: What factors would affect your choice of antibiotic?

Answer: Clarithromycin interacts with simvastatin and the two drugs should not be prescribed together. You could use doxycycline or if this could not be used for any reason the statin should be stopped and only restarted one week after antibiotic treatment is complete.

Classifying ADRs

The ABCDE classification has traditionally been used for ADRs (Whittlesea and Walker 2015). The most common are Types A and B, but it is important to be aware of the other types.

Type A (augmented): These are pharmacologically predictable and dose-dependent. As such, they are common and can be managed by dose reduction. They tend to have a low mortality.

Example: Postural hypotension on initiation of ACE inhibitors. This is why low doses are used initially and titrated up.

Type B (bizarre): These are not pharmacologically predictable or dose dependent. They are uncommon and tend to have a higher incidence of mortality. Discontinuation of the drug is necessary. The causes of these reactions may have an immunological or genetic basis.

Example: Allergic reactions to antibiotics that can lead to anaphylaxis. Also, blood dyscrasias in patients prescribed the antipsychotic clozapine. Patients prescribed this drug are rigorously monitored to identify if they may be developing this ADR. It is still used because it is effective in patients with extremely hard-to-manage conditions who have not responded to other antipsychotics.

Type C (chronic): Mostly associated with chronic use leading to some kind of toxic response.

Example: Suppression of the hypothalamus-pituitary gland-adrenal cortex by long-term systemic glucocorticoid treatment.

Type D (delayed): The time course of developing these kinds of reaction is not necessarily immediate. Reactions can be seen after treatment has ceased.

Example: Drugs prescribed in pregnancy that may cause teratogenesis where the ADR may only become evident after birth. Another example is anticancer drugs that can in fact cause mutagenesis/carcinogenesis and may in fact increase the risk of a secondary malignancy following treatment.

Type E (end of treatment): These reactions occur when treatment is stopped, so include withdrawal reactions and rebound reactions when physiological systems have adapted to the presence of the drug.

Examples: Abruptly ceasing opiates after long-term use can cause withdrawal reactions. Stopping beta-blockers suddenly can cause rebound tachycardia due to upregulation of receptors.

Practical Steps to Minimise ADRs

♦ Make sure you are able to apply knowledge of the pharmacodynamic and pharmacokinetic properties of any drugs you are initiating to your patient.

- Make sure you look carefully at the patient's drug history to look for the potential for any drug interactions that may lead to an ADR, e.g. NSAIDs and SSRIs leading to an increased risk of GI bleed.
- Make sure you ask about any OTC and herbal products, as these can influence the risk of an ADR.
- Consider the patient's medical history and the possibility of an ADR, e.g. starting drugs that cause postural hypotension in a patient at risk of falls.
- Utilise any prescribing support available to you, such as computerised alerts on prescribing systems.
- If there is a risk of an ADR, consider other therapeutic options, e.g. non-pharmacological management or using another class of drug that poses less risk.
- Make sure patients at risk are made aware of warning signs and reviewed regularly.
- In very complex cases, talk to a colleague or pharmacist to help assess the risk/benefit ratio of prescribing and possible options.

Think about:

Developing your knowledge further by working through the Clinical Knowledge Summary (CKS) available on the NICE (n.d.a) website on ADRs. This covers the practical aspects of assessing and managing a reaction, as well as reporting the ADR.

Reporting ADRs

It is vital that all those working in healthcare engage with reporting of ADRs as part of what is called post-marketing surveillance. This means that all drugs are intensively monitored after they come on to the market and any suspected ADRs are reported to the MHRA. These new drugs can be identified in the BNF as they have a black triangle next to the drug name. This black triangle usually stays in place for five years, but this can be extended if there are any concerns about the medication. The reason for this monitoring is that the clinical trials drugs go through before being granted a product licence will only ever identify some of the ADRs that may happen when a patient takes a drug. There are occasions where medicines are withdrawn from the market because ADRs not picked up in the clinical trials were reported in practice by clinicians.

Potential ADRs should be reported to the MHRA via the yellow card scheme. This can be done in a variety of ways, including online. It can also be done by the patient themselves. There are certain criteria about what and when to report. Find out how to do this so that when you have a patient present with an ADR you know what to do.

> ## Think about:
> - Identifying particular drugs or patient groups that you will be encountering that are at high risk of developing ADRs.
> - How you think you will identify and manage ADRs in your area of practice?
> - Do you know what, when and how to report an ADR?
> - Do you know what a black triangle drug is and when you should report these? (If you don't, then go to https://www.gov.uk/drug-safety-update/the-black-triangle-scheme-or to find out.)

Individual Patient Variation: Pharmacogenetics

Not all patients are the same and you will be familiar with this in terms of things such as their medical history or pre-disposition to certain conditions. What you may not be aware of, however, is that the way patients handle drugs can vary depending on genetic factors. The branch of pharmacology that focuses on this is known as pharmacogenetics.

There is significant interest in how this can be used in the future to tailor medicines to patients depending on their genetic makeup. It may well be during your career that this will become part of routine practice. For now, however, it is enough to be aware that genetic variation can affect certain drugs used in practice.

One way is through variable metabolism of drugs. Codeine is one important example of a drug that shows variable metabolism due the genetic profile of the patient. It is metabolised by CYP450 isoform CYP2D6. There is a significant inter-patient variation in the production of this isoform, meaning that the rate of codeine metabolism varies widely between patients. As codeine is a prodrug that is metabolised to the active metabolite morphine, this means that the therapeutic response also varies widely. Patients are categorised by their ability to metabolise codeine as either poor metabolisers or extensive metabolisers:

- **Poor metabolisers of codeine**: Reduced therapeutic effect due to reduced ability to metabolise codeine into morphine.
- **Extensive metabolisers of codeine**: Increased levels of morphine mean there is a risk of adverse effects, such as drowsiness and respiratory depression.

Conclusion

In this chapter, we have covered many different topics and hopefully you now have a greater understanding of the range of ways in which individual patients can respond to medicines differently. Your confidence and ability to tailor treatment will grow with your knowledge and experience. It is important to take the opportunity to focus on any groups that you will be working with during your independent prescribing training. The references and further reading included below will hopefully give you a starting point for building this knowledge and experience. One of the key factors in safe and effective prescribing is knowing where to find the information you need. Making sure you build up an awareness of where to find this information will support you in being as safe and effective as possible when you start out as a prescriber.

Key Points of This Chapter

♦ No patient is the same as another; the skill is to be able to assess the patient in front of you and apply your pharmacology knowledge to that person.

♦ If you know the basic principles of pharmacology, these will help you to identify those patients who may handle drugs differently.

♦ It takes time to build up knowledge and experience of working with specific patient groups, so make sure you invest this time in those areas within your scope of practice.

♦ It is also important to build up your knowledge of where to find the information and support you will need when you initially begin prescribing.

References and Further Reading

Aronson, J. K. (ed.) (2006) *Meyler's Side Effects of Drugs: The International Encyclopedia of Adverse Drug Reactions and Interactions*. Oxford: Elsevier.

Ashley, C. and Dunleavy, A. (2014) *The Renal Drug Handbook: The Ultimate Prescribing Guide for Renal Practitioners*. 4th edn. London: Radcliffe Publishing.

Atkinson, C. and Kirkham, S. (1999) Unlicensed uses for medication in a palliative care unit. *Palliative Medicine* 13: 145–152.

British National Formulary (BNF) *British Medical Association and Royal Pharmaceutical Society of Great Britain*. London: BNF. (Regular updates are published every quarter – make sure you use the most up-to-date edition or use the online version available on the NICE website.)

British National Formulary (BNF) (2020) Prescribing in Palliative Care. *British Medical Association and Royal Pharmaceutical Society of Great Britain*. London: BNF. Available at: https://bnf.nice.org.uk/guidance/prescribing-in-palliative-care.html.

Cahill, P. (2015) Prescribing for patients with multimorbidity: Aiming to tailor to patient-set goals. *British Journal of General Practice* 65(632): 114–115.

Davey, P., Wilcox, M., Irving, W. et al. (2015) Prescribing in special groups: Effects of age, pregnancy, body weight, and hepatic and renal impairment. In *Antimicrobial Chemotherapy*. Oxford: Oxford University Press, pp. 148–158.

Dickman, A. and Schneider, J. (2015) *The Syringe Driver: Continuous Subcutaneous Infusions in Palliative Care*. Oxford: Oxford University Press.

Dodds, L. J. (2013) *Drugs in Use: Clinical Case Studies for Pharmacists*. London: Pharmaceutical Press.

Faull, C., De Caestecker, S., Nicholson, A. and Black, F. (2012) *Handbook of Palliative Care*. Hoboken, NJ: Wiley-Blackwell

Katzung, B., Masters, S. and Trevor, A. (eds) (2012) *Basic and Clinical Pharmacology*. Maidenhead: McGraw-Hill.

Mangoni, A. A. and Jackson, S. H. D. (2004) Age-related changes in pharmacokinetics and pharmacodynamics: Basic principles and practical applications. *British Journal of Clinical Pharmacology* 57(1): 6–14.

National Institute for Clinical Excellence (NICE) (2015) Care of dying adults in the last days of life: NICE guideline [NG31]. Available at: https://www.nice.org.uk/guidance/ng31 (last accessed: 6 December 2019).

National Institute for Clinical Excellence (NICE) (n.d.a) Adverse drug reactions. Available at: https://cks.nice.org.uk/adverse-drug-reactions (last accessed: 6 December 2019).

NHS UKMi (2016) *Medicines Q&A: What Factors Need to Be Considered When Dosing Patients with Renal Impairment*. Q&A 167.6.

Payne, R. A., Abel, G. A., Avery, A. J. et al. (2014) Is polypharmacy always hazardous? A retrospective cohort analysis using linked electronic health records from primary and secondary care. *British Journal of Clinical Pharmacology* 77(6): 1073–1082.

Pirmohamed, M., James, S., Meakin, S. et al. (2004) Adverse drug reactions as cause of admission to hospital: Prospective analysis of 18,820 patients. *British Medical Journal* 329: 15–19.

Preston, C. (ed.) (2016) *Stockley's Drug Interactions*. London: Pharmaceutical Press.

Rang, H. P., Ritter, J. M., Flower, R. J. et al. (2016) *Rang & Dale's Pharmacology*. London: Elsevier.

Smyth J. (ed.) (2015) The NEWT guidelines. Wrexham: Betsi Cadwaladr University Local Health Board (Eastern Division). Available (with a subscription) at: http://www.newtguidelines.com/ (last accessed: 6 December 2019).

Specialist Pharmacy Service (SPS) (2014) What pharmacokinetic and pharmacodynamic factors need to be considered when prescribing drugs for patients with liver disease? Available at: https://www.sps.nhs.uk/articles/what-pharmacokinetic-and-pharmacodynamic-factors-need-to-be-considered-when-prescribing-drugs-for-patients-with-liver-disease-2// (last accessed: 6 December 2019).

Tinetti, M. E., Bogardus, S. T. and Agostini, J. V. (2004) Potential pitfalls of disease-specific guidelines for patients with multiple conditions. *New England Journal of Medicine* 351: 2870–2874.

Todd, J. and Davies, A. (1999) Use of unlicensed medication in palliative medicine. *Palliative Medicine* 13: 446.

Twycross, R., Wilcock, A. and Howard, P. (2018) *Palliative Care Formulary (PCF6)*. London: Pharmaceutical Press. Also available at: medicinescomplete.com.

Walker, R. and Whittlesea C. (eds) (2018) *Clinical Pharmacy and Therapeutics*. Oxford: Elsevier/Churchill Livingstone. (This contains good chapters on pharmacogenetics, ADRs and drug interaction, as well as specific therapeutic areas.)

Weersink, R. A., Bouma, M., Burger, D. M. et al. (2016) Evaluating the safety and dosing of drugs in patients with liver cirrhosis by literature review and expert opinion. *British Medical Journal Open* 6: 1–7.

White, R. and Bradnam, V. (2015) *Handbook of Drug Administration via Enteral Feeding Tubes*. London: Pharmaceutical Press.

World Health Organization (WHO) (1972) International drug monitoring: The role of national centres. WHO Technical Report No. 498. Available at: http://apps.who.int/iris/handle/10665/40968 (last accessed: 6 December 2019).

Useful Websites

Clinical Knowledge Summaries from NICE on different clinical topics that can link to the topics covered in this chapter. Available at: https://cks.nice.org.uk/#?char=A.

The Electronic Medicines Compendium (eMC) is a database of the SPCs for medicines that are licensed in the UK. Available at: https://www.medicines.org.uk/emc.

The MHRA provides information on medicines safety and is particularly useful for reporting of side effects/ADRs. Available at: https://www.gov.uk/government/organisations/medicines-and-healthcare-products-regulatory-agency.

The National Institute for Clinical Excellence (NICE) includes guidance on various topics, such as managing ADRs and prescribing in renal disease. It is important to be aware of what guidance they have that may influence your practice as they are a national NHS body producing evidence-based guidance. Available at: https://www.nice.org.uk.

NHS Specialist Pharmacy Services (SPS) is a website that has useful information on prescribing for staff working in the NHS. There are various articles that review evidence and aim to help prescribing decisions, particularly where there is limited evidence. Available at: https://www.sps.nhs.uk.

Chapter 6

Therapeutics of Conditions Commonly Seen in District Nursing Practice

Jennifer Gorman

In This Chapter

♦ Introduction
♦ Chronic obstructive pulmonary disease
♦ Chronic heart failure
♦ Diabetes mellitus
♦ Managing infections
♦ Pain management
♦ Key points of this chapter
♦ Conclusion
♦ References and further reading.

Introduction

This chapter focuses on some of drugs that are used in conditions commonly seen in district nursing. To cover in the detail the depth that you will need to prescribe for these conditions would require a chapter on each condition. This is intended as an overview from which you can identify areas you need to build your knowledge. There are references and links to websites provided for you to help with this. It is essential to remember that there will be local variations in the prescribing in these therapeutic areas due to differences in local guidance and formularies.

Chronic Obstructive Pulmonary Disease

It is estimated that about 3 million patients suffer with this condition in the UK (Walker and Whittlesea 2018). It is not a disease as such but rather a term that encompasses a range of disorders such as chronic bronchitis and emphysema (Mak 2017). This means that patients present with chronic obstruction of the airways that is poorly reversible. As this is a chronic condition, patients will require medication over the course of many years. Optimising the therapeutic outcome of prescribed medication is essential, due to the profound impact this can have on patients' quality of life. The aim of medication is to improve lung function and reduce exacerbations.

In this section, we will look at the different treatment options, guidance to support prescribing decisions and managing acute exacerbations.

Bronchodilators

Bronchodilators produce their therapeutic action by acting as agonists at beta-2 receptors on bronchial smooth muscle. The drug-receptor interaction causes bronchodilation, reducing bronchospasm. There are two main classes of beta-2 receptor agonists: short-acting bronchodilators (SABAs) and long-acting bronchodilators (LABAs).

SABAs such as salbutamol and terbutaline have a quick action, working within 5–15 minutes of inhalation (Pearce 2012). The effects last about 2–4 hours and generally they are prescribed on a 'when required' (PRN) basis.

LABAs such as salmeterol, indacaterol and formeterol have a 9–12-hour duration (Pearce 2012).

SABAs and LABAs cause side effects that include tachycardia, muscle cramp, fine tremor and hypokalaemia. The side effects are generally pharmacologically predictable due to their activity at beta-2 receptors and are dose related. The most serious side effect is cardiac arrhythmia, which can be caused as a result of drug-induced hypokalaemia. This is only usually seen in patients using particularly high doses and is an important reason for the frequency and dose the patient is using to be monitored regularly.

Anticholinergic Drugs

Muscarinic antagonists are anticholinergic drugs that act as antagonists at muscarinic receptors in the airways responsible for bronchoconstriction. By blocking the activity of these receptors there is relaxation of bronchial muscle. Like bronchodilators, they are available in both short-acting or long-acting forms known as short-acting muscarinic antagonists (SAMAs) and long-acting antimuscarinic antagonists (LAMAs).

The most commonly used SAMA in practice is ipratropium bromide, which comes both as an inhaler and as nebules. It has a maximal effect in 30–60 minutes and the duration of action is 3–6 hours (NICE CKS 2019).

Tiotropium is a LAMA that has been prescribed for many years as maintenance therapy in COPD. Due to its long duration of action it need only be administered once daily. There are various new LAMAs coming on to the market, such as aclidinium, umeclidinium and glycopyrronium, that are also licensed for maintenance treatment in COPD. They are still under intensive surveillance by the MHRA and their place in therapy is still being established (Walker and Whittlesea 2018).

The side effects of these drugs are related to the fact that they can bind to other cholinergic receptor subtypes. This means that they can cause other anticholinergic effects, such as constipation, dry mouth and nausea. Having said that, because they are administered to the lung, there is little systemic absorption and so they are generally well tolerated.

Corticosteroids

Inhaled corticosteroids (ICS) are used as a mainstay of treatment in asthma due to the role of the inflammatory response in the pathology of asthma. Because of the difference in the underlying nature of COPD, they do not have the same role in this condition and they are not prescribed as monotherapy. Their role is more limited and tends to be restricted to more severe disease. This is because the evidence does not show that they improve mortality (NICE CKS 2019). They are used in conjunction with other inhaled treatments as some evidence suggests they improve quality of life and reduce the frequency of exacerbations (Pearce 2012). There is, however, some evidence emerging that they are potentially over-used in COPD patients (Walker and Whittlesea 2018). One trial showed that withdrawing inhaled steroids in patients with severe COPD that was stable did not lead to an increase in exacerbations (Magnussen et al. 2014). It may be that their role in treatment changes in the coming years as more evidence emerges.

It is known that patients with COPD show varied degrees of improvement in lung function in response to ICS. Historically patients underwent reversibility testing prior to initiation of corticosteroids for this reason. Current guidance states that reversibility testing to ICS should not generally be done as it does not predict response to long-term therapy (Brennan 2019).

There is the possibility of both localised and systemic side effects when ICS are prescribed. The most common local side effects are a hoarse voice and candidiasis of the throat and mouth. They are an indicator that there is a problem with the patient's inhaler technique because they are caused by oropharyngeal deposition of the drug. With correct technique, deposition should all be in the lung. High doses of inhaled medication may also lead to systemic effects, and patients should carry steroid cards to alert prescribers that they are on this medication. This should not be stopped suddenly due to the risk of adrenal suppression. There is also the possibility of corticosteroid-induced osteoporosis and pneumonia. NICE guidance states that prescribers should be prepared to discuss the risk of these side effects with patients, including pneumonia (NICE 2018a).

It may be necessary to use oral corticosteroids in some patients, either acutely to manage exacerbations or long term in very severe disease when they cannot be withdrawn after an exacerbation. There are numerous side effects that can be seen with systemic corticosteroids, including adrenal suppression, gastrointestinal disturbance, hyperglycaemia (which can cause diabetes), osteoporosis, hypertension and changes in mental health including psychosis.

Because of the risk of adrenal insufficiency with prolonged steroid use, they must be withdrawn gradually in patients who have (BNF 2019):

♦ Received more than 40 milligrams of prednisolone (or equivalent) daily for more than one week

- Been given repeat doses in the evening
- Received more than three weeks' treatment
- Recently received repeated courses (particularly if taken for longer than three weeks)
- Taken a short course within one year of stopping long-term therapy
- Other possible causes of adrenal suppression.

Patients prescribed steroids may also need alterations to existing medication or additional medications to counteract the problems associated with therapy, e.g. initiation of bone protection in patients using steroids long term to protect against osteoporosis. Enteric-coated medications have been used to reduce GI effects, but there is no clear evidence they are more effective than giving gastric protection with a proton pump inhibitor (Pearce 2012).

Methylxanthines

Theophylline and aminophylline are methylxanthines that are used orally or IV as bronchodilators. They have a narrow therapeutic window and so require therapeutic drug monitoring. They are not used particularly commonly in COPD, as the evidence for their efficacy is not particularly strong and they have poor tolerability (Walker and Whittlesea 2018).

When prescribing these drugs, there needs to be appropriate routine monitoring. There should be additional monitoring if:

- There is a change in dose
- There is a change in the patient's ability to process the medication, such as in liver impairment
- An interacting medication, such as ciprofloxacin or clarithromycin, is started.

Another interaction that is particularly important in patients with COPD is between methylxanthines and smoking. Smoking can increase the clearance of theophylline and may mean that increased doses are required (Nuelin SA 250 milligram SPC, EMC medicines). The single most important step a patient with COPD can take in improving their condition is to stop smoking, and this should be encouraged whenever possible (Walker and Whittlesea 2018). Any patient who is prescribed a methylxanthine must, however, be advised that their dose may need to be adjusted if they stop smoking as there is a risk of toxicity.

Mucolytics

The most commonly prescribed mucolytic used in practice for patients with chronic cough and production of sputum is carbocisteine. The evidence for efficacy is limited and it should only be prescribed for a trial period of 6–8 weeks (Walker and Whittlesea 2018). After this time, the patient should be assessed for signs of clinical improvement. Treatment should be withdrawn if no reduction in sputum production or frequency of cough is seen. Mucolytic drugs should not routinely be offered to prevent exacerbation in patients with stable COPD (NICE 2018a).

Approaches to Treatment in COPD

Figure 6.1 shows the summary of how treatment of COPD is approached based on NICE guidance. Inhaled treatment is started only after preliminary interventions are offered to patients and inhaled treatment is needed to relieve breathlessness or exercise limitation.

Initial management is based on monotherapy with either a SABA or SAMA. This is stepped up if symptoms are not controlled to dual therapy. Triple therapy may be recommended in some patients who still have symptoms or exacerbations despite dual therapy, as it can be effective in reducing both symptoms and exacerbations in these patients (NICE CKS 2019).

Prescribing the most appropriate and cost-effective therapies in COPD patients can be difficult. The choice of treatment is dependent not only on the pharmacological properties of the drug but also on the patient's ability to use the inhaled delivery system effectively. A key element of prescribing in this area is ensuring patients are able to use the devices they are prescribed. There are so many different inhalers on the market, with new ones appearing all the time, but keeping up to date is essential to ensure you are following national and local guidance. Many local areas produce guidance that includes preferred treatment options, information on dosing, guidance on how devices should be used and the cost of treatment. These can be an extremely helpful support when prescribing.

Inhaled Drug Delivery Systems

Formulating medicines into inhaled devices requires a huge amount of time and skill. The particle size contained in the medication is crucial as to whether it will reach the lung or get stuck somewhere in the mouth or throat. When the device is activated, the drug aerosol needs to come out at just the right pressure to make it to the lungs. As well as these formulation issues, there are also patient factors that are crucial in ensuring patients benefit from treatment. There is a huge focus in this area on taking a patient-centred approach to prescribing of the delivery systems. Most patients can develop adequate inhaler technique, but this can only be achieved if they are given training (NICE 2018a).

Summary of Factors to Consider When Prescribing Inhaled Therapy

- Check local guidelines to make sure you are prescribing in line with local formularies.
- Think about the range of devices available and how they work.
- Match respiratory function (ability to inhale at appropriate rate) to the devices, using an in-check device to check which inhalers will be suitable.
- Check the patient's ability to coordinate actuation of the device and inhalation. Think about whether a breath-actuated device or a spacer might be needed.
- Check the patient's previous experience with inhalers to find out if they have any concerns or preferences.

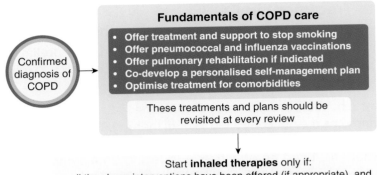

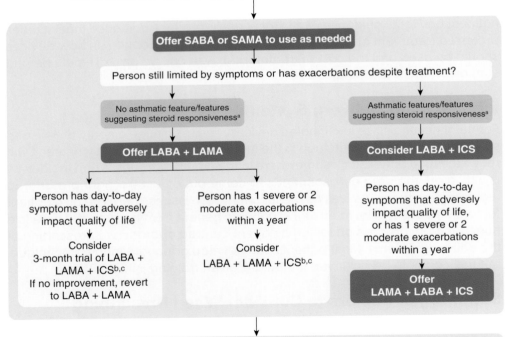

[a]Asthmatic features/features suggesting steroid responsiveness in this context include any previous secure diagnosis of asthma or atopy, a higher blood eosinophil count, substantial variation in FEV1 over time (at least 400 ml) or substantial diurnal variation in peak expiratory flow (at least 20%).

[b]Be aware of an increased risk of side effects (including pneumonia) in people who take ICS.

[c]Document in clinical records the reason for continuing ICS treatment.

Figure 6.1 – Treatment and Management of COPD in over 16s

Source: © NICE (2019). Available from: https://www.nice.org.uk/guidance/ng115/resources/visual-summary-treatment-algorithm-pdf-6604261741.

- Does the patient have any relevant impairment of cognitive function or memory?
- Does the patient have any physical ability/disability issues (e.g. arthritic hands)?
- Make sure that the minimum number of inhalers and the minimum different types of inhaler are prescribed as far as possible. Combination products can be useful but regular review is needed, particularly if they include a high-dose corticosteroid.
- When a selection has been made, ensure the patient has adequate training on the device.
- Check inhaler technique as part of routine practice.

To support patients with the inhaler technique, there are a range of online videos available so that they can practice at home. Community pharmacists can also support patients with their inhaler technique when they are prescribed new inhalers through a service called the New Medicines Service (NMS). If you are not familiar with this service, talk to your local pharmacist as they can offer support to patients who are starting medicines for a range of conditions

Smoking Cessation

It is worth mentioning smoking cessation in this chapter as this is the single most important modifiable factor in slowing the progress of COPD. It can be an incredibly difficult process to manage with your patients. Motivational interviewing can be used to help have a non-judgemental and open conversation with patients about stopping smoking. Once a patient has decided they want help to stop, then pharmacological therapy can be used in conjunction with an appropriate support programme. Evidence-based approaches to stopping smoking include behavioural therapy, as well as pharmacological support through nicotine replacement therapy (NRT), bupropion and varenicline. Varenicline is usually only prescribed as part of a support programme (NICE 2018b).

Turn to **Chapter 11** for more on motivational interviewing.

Think about:

- Will you be prescribing nicotine replacement therapy?
- If so, do you need to spend some time with smoking cessation experts to get some practical experience in using these drugs?
- What stop smoking services are available to you locally, and do you know where to refer or signpost patients to if they want help quitting?
- Are you familiar with Nice Guideline NG92 (2018) Stop smoking interventions and services? If not, visit: https://www.nice.org.uk/guidance/ng92.

Chronic Heart Failure

Chronic heart failure is a common condition affecting approximately 1–2% of the population in developed countries (Ponikowski et al. 2016). The prevalence increases significantly with age and rises to over 10% in patients over 75 years old (Walker and Whittlesea 2018). It is a progressive condition caused by a complex syndrome that arises from the heart acting ineffectively in its function as a circulatory pump. This results in the circulation of blood around the body being inadequate, so tissues do not receive an adequate amount of oxygen and nutrients. Patients suffer with symptoms linked to defects in left ventricular function, the most common being breathlessness, fatigue and ankle swelling. There may be other symptoms linked to inadequate tissue perfusion, venous congestion and disturbance in the balance of water and electrolytes. Accompanying clinical signs include an elevated jugular venous pressure (JVP) and pulmonary oedema. As a chronic condition, its onset is usually gradual and it is difficult to predict how quickly the disease will progress. Generally, the prognosis is poor, but the trajectory of mortality varies considerably between individuals.

The cause of the condition can be due to structural and/or functional cardiac abnormality. There is usually a myocardial abnormality that leads to ventricular dysfunction, but there may also be abnormalities of the valves, pericardium, endocardium, heart rhythm and conduction (Ponikowski et al. 2016). Other common underlying aetiologies that pre-dispose patients to heart failure include hypertension and coronary artery disease. These are important to manage, as well as the heart failure itself (NICE 2018).

Management of Chronic Heart Failure

Historically, the aim of drug treatment in chronic heart failure was management of symptoms. Diuretics were the mainstay of treatment for this reason, as they are useful for managing symptoms (Ponikowski et al. 2016). An improvement in the understanding of the pathophysiology of the condition has meant that treatments now target various physiological systems in an effort to optimise both quality of life and survival rates. As with all chronic conditions that require multiple drug treatments, there is a need for patients to be involved in decisions about treatment. This is particularly important in heart failure as it seems to be a condition poorly understood by the public. Only 3% of patients were able to identify the condition when given a list of symptoms typically associated with heart failure (Walker and Whittlesea 2018). There is a need for patients to be able to self-monitor their symptoms and any adverse effects from their treatment, so provision of information to patients is essential.

In patients with a preserved ejection fraction, no specific treatment is recommended for the heart failure itself, except for symptomatic treatment with diuretics. Underlying pathology of conditions that may worsen the heart failure should be treated as per local and/or national guidance (NICE 2018b).

The treatments outlined below are therefore only indicated in patients with a reduced ejection fraction.

Angiotensin-converting Enzyme (ACE) Inhibitors

These drugs are considered essential in the treatment of chronic heart failure with a reduced ejection fraction. They improve the symptoms of heart failure but also show improved survival (Ponikowski et al. 2016). They act to target some of the compensatory mechanisms that occur in heart failure: arterial and venous vasoconstriction and fluid retention. The renin-angiotensin-aldosterone system is involved in the regulation of cardiac function through various mechanisms, which ACE inhibitors modify.

By inhibition of angiotensin-converting enzyme, they reduce the conversion of angiotensin I to angiotensin II, which is a potent vasoconstrictor. The resulting vasodilation is predominantly arterial but there is also some venous vasodilation (Waller et al. 2014). This leads to a decrease in both preload and afterload. Angiotensin II also stimulates the release of aldosterone, which is involved in regulating Na^+ and H_2O retention. The reduction in aldosterone caused by ACE inhibitors leads to an increased excretion of Na^+ and H_2O. There is consequently a reduced blood volume, which results in a decrease in preload and venous return to the heart (Neal 2016). Because of this improvement in cardiac output and renal perfusion, there is then a further reduction in oedema (Walker and Whittlesea 2018).

In chronic heart failure with a reduced ejection fraction, as well as the physiological changes there is also remodelling of the ventricle. This structural change contributes to a reduction in the efficiency of the ventricular contraction. The improved survival seen with ACE inhibitors is thought to potentially be due to reversal of this remodelling (Waller et al. 2014)

ACE inhibitors are generally well tolerated by most patients. They should, however, be started at low doses because of the risk of hypotension and titrated with blood pressure monitoring. Patients who have renal artery stenosis can develop renal failure if prescribed ACE inhibitors. Because of this and their renal effects, there needs to be careful monitoring of renal function and electrolytes. Patients should have these parameters monitored at baseline and then routinely during treatment or after a dose change (BNF 2019a). One of the most common side effects patients experience with ACE inhibitors is a dry cough. This occurs in 10–30% of patients and is thought to be linked to the fact that ACE inhibitors cause an increase in kinins in the lungs (Rang et al. 2016; Waller et al. 2014). Angioedema can also occur and is thought to be linked to the build-up of bradykinin.

Angiotensin II Receptor Antagonists (ARBs)

This class of drugs is similar in its activity to ACE inhibitors, but instead of reducing the amount of angiotensin II they block the receptor it acts on. They do have the advantage of not producing an accumulation of kinins and are therefore suitable for patients who are intolerant of ACE inhibitors.

Beta-blockers

Beta-blockers in the past were contraindicated in heart failure. Logically this makes sense as they have a negative ionotropic effect, meaning that they reduce the force of the heart's contraction. However, it has been shown that heart failure is associated with a harmful overactivation of the sympathetic nervous system (Walker and Whittlesea 2018). Beta-blockers act to reduce this and it is thought this is the reason why evidence demonstrates they improve long-term survival. Clinical trials have shown that when carvedilol, bisoprolol and metoprolol were prescribed together with an ACE inhibitor and a diuretic for one year, they reduced mortality from 11–17% to 7–12% (Neal 2016). These drugs are recommended in all stable, symptomatic patients with heart failure due to left ventricular dysfunction, unless there is a contraindication, such as in a patient with reversible airway disease. There is evidence to suggest that patients with COPD who have heart failure should be treated with beta-blockers, although they should be introduced with caution and appropriate monitoring should be put in place (Walker and Whittlesea 2018)

Because beta-blockers reduce myocardial contractility, they may make symptoms worse when initiated. To minimise the problems when initiating the drug, low doses are used to begin with and titration occurs slowly over weeks or months (Neal 2016). Patients must be advised that they may feel worse initially and should be given clear guidance on the titration regimen they are being prescribed.

Diuretics

Mineralocorticoid Receptor Antagonists (MRAs)

MRAs are recommended by NICE in addition to ACE inhibitors and beta-blockers in patients whose symptoms are not controlled with dual therapy. This class blocks aldosterone at the mineralocorticoid receptor and provide another mechanism through which to block the renin-angiotensin-aldosterone system. They have been shown in clinical trials to reduce both mortality and hospital admission (Pitt 2017). Electrolytes and renal function need to be monitored before and after initiation along with when there is any dose change.

Diuresis is used to treat the symptoms associated with pulmonary and peripheral oedema (Ponikowski et al. 2016). This is achieved by blocking the reabsorption of Na^+ in the proximal tubule of the kidneys, where it is usually reabsorbed along with H_2O. Thiazides have a limited action because they have a 'low ceiling'. This means that maximal diuresis is achieved at low doses. They also cause adverse metabolic effects and are ineffective in patients with moderate to severe renal impairment. Loop diuretics are therefore usually the first choice of diuretic in symptomatic heart failure. They are known as 'high ceiling' diuretics, as increasing doses continue to produce increasing diuresis.

In practice, there is a balance in controlling symptoms, with the potential for adverse effects caused by profound diuresis, such as hypovolemia, postural hypotension, electrolyte disturbance and renal failure. Doses of diuretics are usually prescribed in the morning for the practical reasons around increased urine production. This means that the patient can be free to go out after the diuresis has occurred and sleep is not disturbed. It is important to discuss timing with patients, however, as some patients have particular social and lifestyle needs that do not fit with morning dosing and it may be that a timing can be agreed that fits with them better.

Drugs Used Under Specialist Direction

The NICE treatment summary for chronic heart failure in **Figure 6.2** shows that all other drugs used in heart failure should be initiated after specialist reassessment of the patient. You may come across these drugs prescribed in your patient, so it is useful to understand their use. You can find more information in the BNF and the SPC for each drug. There are also links to textbooks and treatment guidelines at the end of the chapter.

Sacubitril/valsartan: This drug is a neprilysin inhibitor. It acts on endogenous peptides and results ultimately in a decrease in the activity of the renin-angiotensin-aldosterone system (Walker and Whittlesea 2018). It has been shown to reduce mortality when used in combination with the ARB valsartan in patients who are not well controlled with ACE inhibitors. Because (like ACE inhibitors) it inhibits the breakdown of bradykinin, there is an increased risk of angioedema if both drugs are given together. The ACE inhibitor should therefore be stopped 36 hours before sacubitril is initiated. This drug is still under intensive post-marketing surveillance and is a new class of medication. It is therefore only recommended for use under specialist advice (SHIFT 2010).

Ivabradine: Ivabradine has negative chronotropic properties, which means it reduces the heart rate. Unlike beta-blockers, however, it does not have negative ionotropic properties and has no effect on the force of the heart's contraction. This means that it slows the heart rate but not the force of contraction. As the effect of the drug is via the sinoatrial node in the heart, the drug is only effective when the patient is in sinus rhythm. There is also a risk of bradycardia when it is added to beta-blocker treatment and so patients should have a heart rate of more than 75 bpm for the drug to be started. Treatment has been shown to be effective in patients with moderate to severe heart failure and so it is not used in mild heart failure.

Nitrates/hydralazine: Nitrates are vasodilators and help to reduce preload. They are often used with hydralazine, which reduces afterload. The use of these drugs has been shown to reduce mortality, but not to the same extent as ACE inhibitors. They are therefore usually reserved for use in patients who are unable to tolerate or who have a contraindication to ACE inhibitors. The reduction in mortality is, however, more pronounced in patients of African descent and so the combination may be used in this patient group (NICE 2018b; Ponikowski et al. 2016).

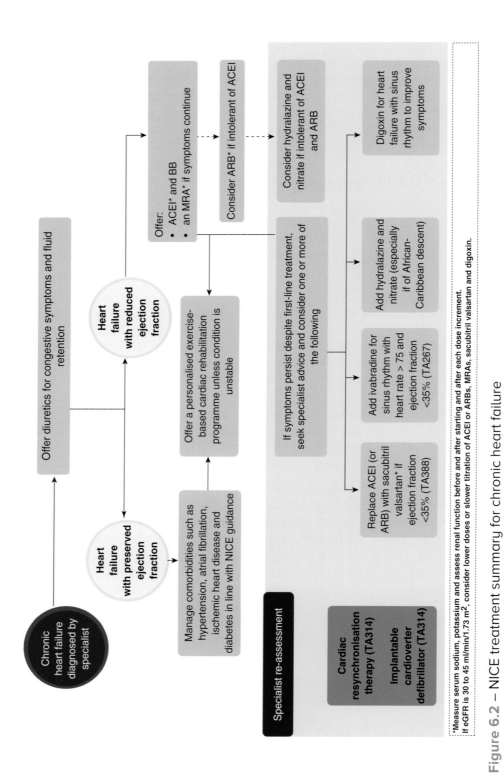

Figure 6.2 – NICE treatment summary for chronic heart failure

Source: © NICE (2018b). Available from: https://www.nice.org.uk/guidance/ng106/resources/chronic-heart-failure-management-visual-summary-pdf-6663137725.

Digoxin: This drug has a positive ionotropic effect and increases the force of the heart's contraction. It has been shown to reduce hospital admissions, but not to reduce mortality. For this reason, it may be used to improve symptoms as an add-on therapy, but not before other therapies have been considered (Walker and Whittlesea 2018). It has only been shown to be an effective treatment for patients who are in sinus rhythm. The drug has a narrow therapeutic window and requires therapeutic drug monitoring. Patients should have serum concentrations monitored as per local guidance and be monitored clinically for signs and symptoms of adverse effects. Toxicity can be exacerbated by electrolyte disturbances and so electrolytes should be monitored. This is particularly important as this group of patients may well be taking diuretics that can lead to electrolyte disturbances.

Optimising Therapy

It is important to optimise therapy in patients with heart failure, with a view to improving symptoms and reducing mortality. One aspect of this is reviewing therapy in patients and ensuring that the choice of drug and dose has been optimised. It is also important to ensure that non-pharmacological interventions, such as lifestyle changes, have been addressed. This means discussing diet, exercise, alcohol intake and smoking with patients. Any underlying factors that can worsen the condition should be optimally managed, e.g. hypertension and atrial fibrillation. Patients should have routine review of all the drugs they are prescribed to ensure there are none that should be avoided in heart failure. For example, NSAIDs promote sodium retention and pose an increased risk of renal impairment, so should be avoided. Remember to advise patients to be careful when buying medicines over the counter (OTC) and to ask their pharmacist if the medication is safe to use. Herbal remedies should also be used with caution and advice should be sought. The SIGN (2016) guidance on managing heart failure has a useful appendix, including some advice on herbal remedies. It is also important if you are prescribing for a patient with heart failure, even if it is for a totally different condition, to ensure there will be no drug interactions.

As with any chronic treatment, prescribers need to regularly check adherence to treatment, symptom control and whether the patient's treatment goals are being met. For example, it may be that the patient's symptoms are not being controlled as well as they would like because they are not following their treatment plan. This could be due to an adverse effect or simply because they are forgetting to take medication. It may be that a simple adjustment of the timing or formulation of a medication could be all that is needed to improve symptom control.

Another important factor in optimising treatment is working as part of the multidisciplinary team (MDT). This may involve referring patients to heart failure specialists or working with them once a patient is discharged. NICE (2018b) guideline NG106 goes into more detail about the role of the MDT in managing heart failure patients and, if you are going to be prescribing for these patients, you should be familiar with this guidance.

Turn to **Chapter 11** for more on optimising medicines, including how to identify intentional and non-intentional non-adherence.

Diabetes Mellitus

Diabetes mellitus is a metabolic condition where there is chronic hyperglycaemia caused by either a relative or total absence of insulin, which may be combined with insulin resistance. This has a variety of consequences, including circulating glucose not being taken up into tissues, such as the muscle, liver and adipose tissue. As a consequence, the body tries to remove excess circulating glucose in the urine, causing glycosuria, which leads to polyuria due to the resulting osmotic diuresis. The patient then becomes dehydrated and so becomes thirsty and drinks excessively (polydipsia). Another consequence is that, since the body is starved of glucose as a source of energy, proteins and fats are broken down instead. In type 1 diabetes this can lead to the emergency situation of diabetic ketoacidosis (DKA). Because type 2 diabetics tend to have some residual insulin production in the pancreas, DKA does not usually occur in this group of patients. This is because the body can normally still produce enough energy through glucose metabolism to avoid this emergency reaction.

There are various long-term complications of diabetes that occur as a result of the metabolic imbalances seen. These are particularly associated with complications linked to large (macrovascular) and small (microvascular) blood vessels. Macrovascular complications are responsible for 75% of deaths related to diabetes (Whittlesea and Walker 2018). Careful management of the condition is needed to prevent complications.

Macrovascular complications:

♦ **Cardiovascular disease**, which can lead to hypertension and ischaemic heart disease.
♦ **Cerebrovascular disease**, which can lead to stroke.

Microvascular complications:

♦ **Nephropathy**, which can lead to microalbuminuria, macroalbuminuria and renal failure.
♦ **Peripheral neuropathy**, which can lead to loss of peripheral sensation (e.g. in the feet), pain and ulceration.
♦ **Retinopathy**, which can lead to visual impairment.
♦ **Autonomic neuropathy**, which can lead to impotence.

Type 2 diabetes is the most common form of diabetes and accounts for about 90% of cases in the West (Waller et al. 2014). The condition is becoming increasingly prevalent, with the number of patients with diabetes rising by 53% between 2006 and 2013 (Whittlesea and Walker 2018).

Drugs Used to Treat Type 1 and Type 2 Diabetes

Although diabetes is broken down in to two subtypes, it is currently uncertain whether they are two distinct diseases or different manifestations of the same disease process (Waller et al. 2014). As the underlying pathology of the types varies, there are important differences between approaches to treating the two patient groups. In type 1 patients there is destruction of the pancreatic cells that produce insulin, caused by an autoimmune reaction. This absence of pancreatic cells capable of producing insulin is why type 1 used to be known as insulin-dependent diabetes. In type 2 diabetes, dietary changes and oral treatments are often able to maintain patients' glycaemic control initially. This is because in the early stages of the disease, resistance to insulin develops. This is often because patients are overweight, which leads to an increase in cellular insulin resistance. This resistance means that less glucose is taken up into tissues, but there is usually sufficient insulin being secreted from pancreatic cells to overcome the resistance. As the condition develops, however, there is a relative reduction in insulin secretion. This means that eventually patients may end up requiring insulin to ensure adequate glycaemic control.

Insulin Therapy

Insulin is the first-line treatment in type 1 diabetes and is also used in type 2 diabetes when other agents have proved unsuccessful. Because insulin is a protein, it cannot be given orally as it would be digested before being absorbed. It is therefore injected subcutaneously. The rate of absorption following administration can be adjusted by increasing the particle size or complexing it with another particle, such as zinc or protamine (Neal 2016). The rationale for this is to mirror as much as possible the physiological release of insulin. Normally there is a basal level of insulin circulating that allows utilisation of glucose through the day. When food is ingested there is a release of insulin that allows the body to deal with the increased levels of glucose. Patients therefore use a regimen of injections using a mixture of long-acting and short-acting insulins to replicate this. There are several different regimens and the one that is chosen needs to be tailored to the patient.

Basal Bolus Regimen

This is the preferred regimen because it the closest to normal physiology. The basal insulin is provided by a long-acting insulin analogue, such as insulin glargine or detemir. This absorbs slowly and is administered either once or twice daily. The bolus part of the regimen is provided by administration of a short-acting insulin at mealtimes. Short-acting insulins have historically been soluble solutions of insulins that have an onset of action of about 30 minutes, so need to be injected 30 minutes before meals. There are also now insulin analogues, such as insulin lispro, aspart and glulsine. These are recommended for initiation in new patients, having a faster onset and shorter duration than soluble insulins. They can be injected just before a meal. The dose of short-acting insulin can be adjusted depending on the carbohydrate intake and also taking into account anything, such as exercise, that can increase metabolic needs.

Twice-daily Regimen

Some patients find it difficult to manage the basal bolus regimen due to the number of injections required. In these patients, biphasic mixtures can be used, which contain a short-acting element with a longer-acting element that is intended to mimic basal insulin. This obviously does not mimic naturally occurring insulin release as closely as the basal bolus regimen. As the proportions of insulin are fixed, there is also less possibility of adjusting it to the metabolic requirements of the patient. For patients who have a relatively stable lifestyle and cannot manage the basal bolus, it is a useful alternative.

Continuous Subcutaneous Insulin Infusion (CSII or Insulin Pump) Therapy

For patients with type 1 diabetes who have persistently unstable blood glucose levels despite optimised insulin treatment, continuous infusions may be considered by diabetes specialists. For more information on these devices, see NICE technology appraisal 151 (NICE 2008).

Oral Antidiabetic Drugs

Oral drugs used in diabetes act to augment the sensitivity of cells to insulin and promote secretion of insulin. They are therefore only usually used in type 2 diabetes.

Biguanides

Metformin is a biguanide and it is the cornerstone of type 2 diabetes management. It has been used successfully for many years and there is a significant body of evidence that supports it as first-line treatment in this patient group, because of reduction in cardiac mortality and improved lifespan (Neal 2016). It does not affect insulin secretion so does not usually cause hypoglycaemia. It can supress the appetite and therefore causes less weight gain than sulphonylureas, making it a particularly good choice in overweight patients. NICE guidance states that metformin should be continued even if the patient ends up requiring insulin therapy, due the benefit treatment can provide (NICE 2015a).

Gastrointestinal (GI) side effects can be a cause for patients to stop treatment. The problem is usually transient, but to reduce the likelihood of these side effects occurring, the drug should be initiated at 500 milligrams once daily and titrated slowly according to response. See the BNF and the SPC for full details on titrating the dose. There is also a sustained release preparation that can be used to reduce GI upset. Other possible side effects include a metallic taste and decreased vitamin B_{12} absorption.

Lactic acidosis is a rare but potentially fatal side effect that can occur if patients with renal impairment are prescribed metformin. Patients should have eGFR monitored regularly and treatment should be stopped if eGFR is less than 45 ml/min/1.73 m².

Sulphonylureas

This class of drug causes insulin to be secreted from pancreatic islet cells, meaning there needs to be some partially functioning cells for the drugs to be effective. It also means that they can cause hypoglycaemia. Drugs which have a longer half-life have a greater risk, so shorter-acting drugs like gliclazide and glipizide are normally tried first-line. Longer-acting drugs, like glibenclamide, pose a particular risk in the elderly and in patients with renal impairment. In these patients, long-acting drugs should be avoided.

Suphonylureas stimulate the appetite and patients are likely to gain weight with treatment, unless dietary restrictions are followed. This is a major concern with treatment in patients who are already overweight.

Dipeptidyl Peptidase 4 Inhibitors (DPP-4 Inhibitors) or Gliptins

This class of drugs includes linagliptin, sitagliptin, saxagliptin and vildagliptin. Through inhibition of the enzyme DPP-4, they lower blood glucose. This is because DPP-4 is responsible for the inactivation of the incretin hormones GLP-1 and GIP. The incretins are involved in regulating insulin synthesis and secretion and the increased levels of incretins lead to increased insulin synthesis and secretion.

These drugs are weight neutral and generally well tolerated by patients. However, because of the lack of long-term data, particularly on outcomes, they are currently not first-line and are used in combination with other drugs for treating type 2 diabetes.

Pioglitazone

Pioglitazone is the only remaining thiazolidinedione still available on the market, as the other drugs in this class have been withdrawn due to serious hepatic and cardiac toxicity. It does improve HbA1c, but causes weight gain and fluid retention. It also increases the risk of heart failure, bladder cancer and bone fractures (NICE 2015a). Patients should have any pre-disposing risk factors, such as age, assessed before starting treatment. The MHRA (2011) suggests that patients initiated on therapy should be reassessed after 3–6 months to ensure that only patients deriving benefit from treatment continue on the drug.

Sodium-glucose Cotransporter 2 Inhibitors (SGLT2)

This class of drug causes increased urinary excretion of glucose by inhibiting the sodium-glucose cotransporter 2 (SGLT2) in the kidney. It does not cause hypoglycaemia and patients taking these drugs usually have modest weight loss (Waller et al. 2014). There are NICE technology appraisals on dapagliflozin, canagliflozin and empagliflozin that provide information on how they should be used in practice. This class of drug have been associated with serious, life-threatening DKA both during treatment and shortly after stopping. Because of this, the MHRA states that ketones should be tested for, even if blood glucose appears normal, if patients have symptoms of DKA (MHRA 2016).

As glucose is being excreted via the urinary system, there is an increased risk of UTI and genital infection in patients treated with these drugs.

Other Parenteral Therapy: Glucagon-like Peptide-1 (GLP-1) Mimetics

Exenatide and liraglutide are GLP-1 mimetics and act to mimic the incretin hormone GLP-1 by acting as agonists at GLP-1 receptors. This leads to an increase in glucose-dependent synthesis of insulin and the release of insulin from pancreatic cells.

Unlike insulin, they promote weight loss and are particularly useful as an alternative to insulin in patients with type 2 diabetes who are obese. Their use is clinical practice is reserved for specific patient groups, such as those with a BMI >35kgm^2. For full details, see the NICE algorithm on treating type 2 diabetes (NICE 2015a) (Figure 6.3).

Approaches to Treatment in Type 2 Diabetes

A key therapeutic task when working with diabetic patients is agreeing treatment outcomes and sharing prescribing decisions. The first step in this is agreeing a target HbA1c with patients. Ideally the aim of treatment should be to achieve levels of blood glucose that are as near as possible to the normal ranges seen in non-diabetic patients. Usually a target of 48 mmol/mol is recommended in patients on a single therapy that is not associated with hypoglycaemia (NICE 2015a). This may not be realistic or achievable in all patients, however, and if levels rise to 58 mmol/mol or greater, patients should be given advice on lifestyle, diet and medication adherence. The patient should be supported to reach a target of 53 mmol/mol and drug treatment intensified. There may also be the risk that treatment will cause hypoglycaemia if treatment includes those drugs associated with hypoglycaemia. This can be of particular concern in the elderly, who are at risk of falls, or in people who drive/operate machinery. In these patients HbA1c targets may be relaxed. Targets may also be adjusted where it is unlikely that the risk-reduction achieved will be long term, for example in patients with significant co-morbidity or reduced life expectancy.

Treatment in this condition has a large non-pharmacological element to it. Patients need support on adjusting their lifestyle, including advice on nutrition,

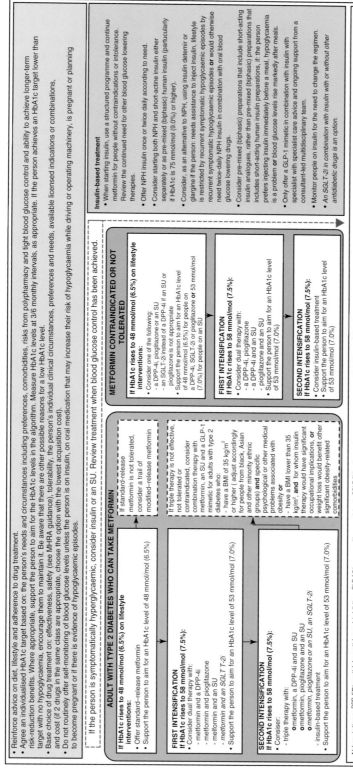

Figure 6.3 – Algorithm for treatment in adults with type 2 diabetes

Source: © NICE (2015a). Available from: https://www.nice.org.uk/guidance/ng28/resources/algorithm-for-blood-glucose-lowering-therapy-in-adults-with-type-2-diabetes-pdf-2185604173.

exercise, smoking and alcohol intake. It is helpful to know where you can signpost patients to locally for further support with this, as it can take a lot of input to help patients make significant changes. Structured educational support programmes have been shown to help patients with some of these aspects. One such programme is the DESMOND type 2 diabetes education programme, but you may have others locally.

If management by diet and exercise alone does not maintain HbA1c levels below the patient's agreed target, then pharmacological treatment should be initiated. Figure 6.3 summarises the stepwise approach to managing type 2 diabetes in NICE (2015a) guidance NG28. The key factors that need to be taken into account when prescribing are:

♦ Drug effectiveness
♦ Drug safety (refer to MHRA safety alerts)
♦ Clinical circumstances of the patient (for example, do they have any relevant co-morbidities)
♦ Patient preferences and agreed treatment outcomes
♦ Tolerability
♦ Cost (if there are two drugs that are equally effective, choose the cheaper of the two).

Management of Other Conditions Associated with Diabetes

In this section, it is not possible to cover all the elements involved in managing the ongoing care of diabetic patients as well as glycaemic control. Diabetic patients are at a higher risk of a whole range of complications and this needs to be taken into account when providing holistic care. Patients who are diabetic and have hypertension, for example, have a much higher risk of both microvascular and macrovascular complications. This means that there are slightly different guidelines for managing hypertension in this group. These patients also have increased risk of renal impairment and it is important that the impact any renal impairment could have on dosing and drug choice is considered when prescribing. Patients should also be advised to consult their pharmacist when buying medicines OTC for these reasons.

Managing Infections

Since the 1940s, there has been a revolution in how infections can be managed. The widespread availability of antibiotics since that time has led to a huge reduction in both the morbidity and mortality associated with infections. Most healthcare workers, however, are increasingly aware that these precious drugs should not be used unwisely. Using antibiotics responsibly is, in fact, one of the most important priorities in modern medicine, because of increasing resistance to these drugs. The World Health Organization (WHO) says that antibiotic resistance is one of the biggest threats to global health today (WHO 2018).

Anyone involved in prescribing to manage infections should therefore be aware of antimicrobial stewardship. This is defined by NICE as: an organisational or healthcare system-wide approach to promoting and monitoring judicious use of antimicrobials to preserve their future effectiveness (NICE 2015b). Most local areas use various ways to encourage antimicrobial stewardship, such as local prescribing guidelines, patient information on using antibiotics responsibly and monitoring prescribing data.

 Turn to **Chapter 7** for more on monitoring of prescribing data.

Principles of Antimicrobial Treatment

One of the reasons for widespread antimicrobial resistance is the inappropriate use of antibiotic drugs. This can be because antibiotics are used to treat infections that do not have a bacterial cause, such as viral infections like the common cold. It can also be because the wrong choice of antibiotic is used. Antimicrobial prescribing guidelines have been developed to support prescribing to try and ensure the right drug is used at the right time for the right patient. It is useful to understand some of the principles that underpin how these guidelines are developed and why recommendations are made.

Empirical Therapy

When antibiotics are needed, guidelines often suggest they are initiated as empirical therapy. This means that the choice is not based on cultures and sensitivities but on clinical diagnosis. This diagnosis allows the choice of antibiotic to be made based on the knowledge of the most likely infecting organism. This is because different bacteria tend to colonise different sites in the body. For example, we know that E. coli is the bacteria most commonly associated with UTIs. First-line antibiotics are therefore those that can act on this group of gram-negative bacteria. In contrast, skin infections are usually linked to gram-positive bacteria, such as staphylococcus. Flucloxacillin acts on staphylococcus and is usually the first-line choice for simple skin infections in patients who are not penicillin allergic.

To ensure empirical therapy gives us the 'best guess' treatment, clinical assessment and diagnosis must be as accurate as possible. This means taking a thorough history and using the most up-to-date, evidence-based screening tools to support diagnosis. It also means that regular review of the patient is done to make sure that treatment is working.

Cultures and Sensitivities

Whilst treatment is often initiated using an empirical approach, it is important that cultures and sensitivities are taken at the right time. This means that if the infection is caused by a bacterium that is resistant to multiple antibiotics or an uncommon pathogen, the information is available to guide treatment. All too often in the past, a second course of treatment has been prescribed which is not based on any data. This risks exposing the patient to more antibiotics that may not be effective and to which they can then demonstrate resistance. Ensure you are familiar with guidance on what samples need to be taken and when, for your patients, when you become a prescriber. Remember that guidance changes all the time, so think about how you will keep up to date.

Spectrum of Activity of Antibiotics

The spectrum of activity of an antibiotic relates to the range of bacteria that the drug can be toxic to. Narrow-spectrum drugs act on a small range of bacteria. Flucloxacillin is an example of a narrow spectrum antibiotic as it acts only on certain gram-positive bacteria. Co-amoxiclav is a penicillin, like flucloxacillin, but it has a broad spectrum of activity. To minimise resistance, we need to try and target only the bacteria that are causing the infection. If we know that an infection is likely to be caused by staphylococcus and we have an antibiotic that only acts on staphylococcus, then we should use that antibiotic. Sometimes it can be more difficult to be sure what the cause is, or it may be likely that there are several types of bacteria causing the infection. This is why broad-spectrum antibiotics like co-amoxiclav are usually reserved for complicated or serious infections.

Mechanism of Action and Pharmacology of the Drug

Antibiotics act by interfering with the normal functioning of some aspect of the bacteria that they target. To minimise the effect that they have on the cells of the human body, they interfere selectively with structural or functional parts of the bacteria that demonstrate differences to human cells. The mechanism of action of penicillins, for example, is by interfering with the bacterial cell wall, because this contains peptidoglycan, a protein not present in human cell walls. Bacterial metabolism can also be targeted; trimethoprim inhibits the enzyme dihydrofolate reductase. The drug is effective even though this enzyme is present in human cells because the functioning of the bacterial enzyme is affected by the presence of lower concentrations of trimethoprim than the human version (Waller et al. 2014). For these effects to be seen, however, the drug needs to actually reach the site of infection at sufficient concentrations to treat the infection. We therefore need to go back to the principles covered in **Chapter 4** with ADME: absorption, distribution, metabolism and elimination. Anything that affects these parameters can impact on the efficacy of the antibiotic. Thinking about treatment of UTIs as an example, we may have a drug that is very effective at killing E. coli *in vitro,* but if it does not concentrate in the urinary system at sufficient levels, it will not treat a UTI.

Antimicrobial Prescribing Guidelines

Local areas will all have their own antimicrobial guidelines, which should be referred to as there may be local variations in resistance. They will also reflect local policies and procedures for other aspects of treatment, such as referral criteria and taking of cultures and sensitivities. It may be that national guidelines are adopted locally if it is assessed that they reflect local needs. Figure 6.4 is an example of a NICE antimicrobial prescribing guideline visual summary, in this case for UTIs. It shows a flow chart decision aid on assessing whether to prescribe, and when to send urine samples and referral criteria. In the full guideline there is also information on what drug to prescribe for different clinical scenarios. There are a whole range of these available on the NICE website focusing on commonly seen infections.

Delayed or Back-up Prescribing

One way of dealing with the uncertainty of whether an infection is self-limiting or needs an antibiotic is by using delayed or back-up prescribing. The patient can be given a prescription that is post-dated, or alternatively given instructions on what clinical criteria would make it appropriate for them to get the drug dispensed. A patient may, for example, be told to start taking the antibiotic if there is no improvement in their condition within 48 hours. It is therefore essential that patients have very clear instructions on why they are being given a delayed prescription and what to do with it.

Because of this, when using back-up (delayed) antibiotic prescribing, patients should be offered:

♦ Reassurance that antibiotics are not needed immediately because they are likely to make little difference to symptoms and may have side effects (for example, diarrhoea, vomiting and rash)
♦ Advice about how to recognise whether they need to use the antimicrobials, and if so:
  ▶ how to get them
  ▶ when to start taking or using them
  ▶ how to take or use them.
♦ Advice about what to do if their condition does not improve despite taking the delayed prescription.

There is a NICE quality statement associated with delayed prescribing in Antimicrobial Stewardship: Quality Standard [QS121] (NICE 2016b).

Resources That Can Be Used with Patients

One way of improving communication with patients about antibiotics is by using resources to support your consultations. This can provide a standardised written source of information that can back up your advice. An example is shown in Figure 6.5, which helps provide advice and reassurance, the normal

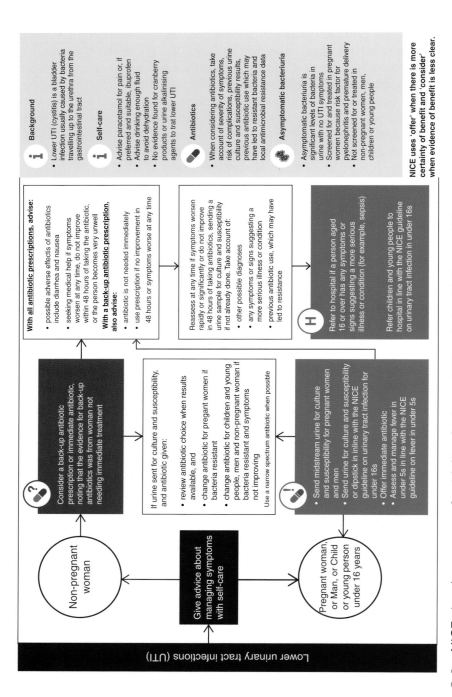

Figure 6.4 – NICE visual summary of guideline for lower UTI antimicrobial prescribing

Source: © NICE (2018c). Available from: https://www.nice.org.uk/guidance/ng109/resources/visual-summary-pdf-6544021069.

Patient name | It is recommended that you self-care

Your infection	Most are better by	How to look after yourself and your family	When to get help
Middle-ear infection	8 days	• Have plenty of rest. • Drink enough fluids to avoid feeling thirsty. • Ask your local pharmacist to recommend medicines to help your symptoms or pain (or both). • Fever is a sign the body is fighting the infection and usually gets better by itself in most cases. You can use paracetamol if you or your child are uncomfortable as a result of a fever. • Use a tissue and wash your hands well to help prevent spread of your infection to your family, friends and others you meet. • Other things you can do suggested by GP or nurse:	**The following are possible signs of serious illness and should be assessed urgently:** 1. If your skin is very cold or has a strange colour, or you develop an unusual rash. 2. If you feel confused or have slurred speech or are very drowsy. 3. If you have difficulty breathing. Signs that suggest breathing problems can include: • breathing quickly • turning blue around the lips and the skin below the mouth • skin between or above the ribs getting sucked or pulled in with every breath. 4. If you develop a severe headache and are sick. 5. If you develop chest pain. 6. If you have difficulty swallowing or are drooling. 7. If you cough up blood. 8. If you are feeling a lot worse.
Sore throat	7–8 days		
Sinusitis	14–21 days		
Common cold	14 days		**If you or your child has any of these symptoms, are getting worse or are sicker than you would expect(even if your/their temperature falls), trust your instincts and seek medical advice urgently from NHS 111 or your GP. If a child under the age of 5 has any of symptoms 1–3 go to A&E immediately or call 999.**
Cough or bronchitis	21 days		**Less serious signs that can usually wait until the next available appointment:** 9. If you are not starting to improve a little by the time given in the 'Most are better by' column. 10. In children with middle-ear infection: if fluid is coming out of their ears or if they have new deafness. 11. Mild side effects such as diarrhea, however seek medical attention if you're concerned. 12. Other ....
Other infection:	...... days		

Back-up antibiotic prescription to be collected after ☐ **days only if you are not starting to feel a little better or you feel worse.**

Collect from: ☐ **Pharmacy** ☐ **General practice reception** ☐ **GP, nurse, other**

• Colds, most coughs, sinusitis, ear infections, sore throats, and other infections often get better without antibiotics, as you body can usually fight these infections on its own.
• Taking antibiotics encourages bacteria that live inside you to become resistant. That means that antibiotics may not work when you really need them.
• Antibiotics can cause side effects such as rashes, thrush, stomach pains, diarrhea, reactions to sunlight, other symptoms, or being sick if you drink alcohol with metronidazole.
• Find out more about how you can make better use of antibiotics and help keep this vital treatment effective by visiting www.nhs.uk/keepantibioticsworking.

Figure 6.5 – Patient information on treating a respiratory tract infection

Source: Public Health England, 2019. Available at: https://campaignresources.phe.gov.uk/resources/campaigns/58/resources/2133.

course length of a respiratory tract infection, what self-care can be done and when to get help. It also provides information about delayed prescribing if this is deemed appropriate. There are a range of these leaflets and other resources that support antimicrobial stewardship on the Royal College of General Physicians (RCGP) website as part of the TARGET (Treat Antibiotics Responsibly, Guidance, Education, Tools) antibiotic toolkit. For more information go to https://www.rcgp.org.uk/targetantibiotics.

Patient Factors When Prescribing Antibiotics

There are a range of patient factors that need to be considered in conjunction with guidelines when deciding on treatment. Drug-drug interactions are one factor that should be considered. Doxycycline interacts with iron preparations, leading to a significant reduction in the absorption of doxycycline, which can lead to treatment failure. Patients should be advised to separate taking the doses of these two drugs as much as possible. Drug-patient interactions can also occur; tetracyclines should be avoided in children and pregnancy because permanent discolouration of the teeth can occur.

Another important patient factor is any allergy that the patient has to antibiotics. The first thing to consider is the nature of the allergy and to try to differentiate between a true allergy and an intolerance. If the patient has had an anaphylactic reaction, they should never be exposed to the class of antibiotic to which they had that reaction. You also need to be cautious

Case Study 6.1

To develop your knowledge and skills, think about a patient you have seen in practice with an infection and answer the following questions:

1. What is the site of infection and the likely infecting organism?
2. What drug acts on the organism and can it reach sufficient concentrations at the site of infection?
3. What route and formulation will optimise the concentration at the site of infection?
4. Are there any local patterns of resistance to drugs commonly used to treat this infection?
5. Are there any patient factors that could alter the likely effectiveness e.g. renal or liver impairment, co-morbidities, drug interactions or previous courses of antibiotics?
6. What other considerations are there, such as source control, ensuring regular reviews and obtaining cultures and sensitivities at an appropriate time?

about whether there is the possibility of cross-sensitivity to other classes of antibiotics. Patients may have a documented allergy to an antibiotic but, when questioned, they actually only suffered from an upset stomach or diarrhoea. This would be classed as an intolerance rather than an allergy. It is important that as a prescriber, you ask about the nature of the ADR that the patient has and ensure that this is documented correctly. If a patient at some point has a life-threatening infection and an antibiotic is withheld because they have an allergy documented which in fact was only an intolerance, it could have a huge clinical impact.

Pain Management

Pain can be challenging to manage, as it is a complex phenomenon which is very subjective. There are a range of factors that can influence the extent to which the patient experiences suffering because of the sensation of pain. It is a sensation that arises initially in response to some noxious stimulus, for example as a result of an injury. This acute pain is also known as nociceptive pain and usually resolves once the underlying stimulus, such as the injury, is resolved. In some cases, however, pain can become chronic and outlasts the resolution of the initial stimulus. This is due to changes in the way that the nociceptive neuronal pathways function and leads to what is known as neuropathic pain. Because of the differences in the underlying pathology, a different approach to treating nociceptive and neuropathic pain has developed. It is important to understand, however, that depending on the origin of the pain there can be a mixture of nociceptive and neuropathic elements, and so some patients may require treatments that target both types of pain.

Analgesic Drugs

Below is a brief summary of the key analgesic drugs. To develop your knowledge of the pharmacology and therapeutics of any of these drugs, explore some of the further reading at the end of the chapter.

Paracetamol: This is a drug that is commonly used by patients at home as it is widely accessible OTC. It is a suitable first-line choice for most patients presenting with mild-to-moderate pain. It resembles an NSAID, but produces only an analgesic and antipyretic effect and not an anti-inflammatory effect (Rang et al. 2016). The advantage of this is that paracetamol does not have some of the adverse effects that can be seen with NSAIDs, such as GI irritation and sodium and fluid retention.

NSAIDs: These drugs reduce inflammation and are therefore useful in pain associated with inflammatory conditions. They are, however, well known to have a range of side effects, such as gastric ulceration and bleeding, sodium retention and renal impairment. In some asthmatic patients they can precipitate bronchospasm. Care must therefore be taken in assessing patients for their suitability and you must be familiar with the cautions and contraindications for this class of drugs. Generally, the advice is that they are used for the shortest possible time at the lowest possible dose. For more information on assessing the suitability of patients, see NICE (2015c).

Opioids: These drugs act on neuronal pathways involved in the transmission of pain from the periphery to the CNS (Waller et al. 2014). They are generally effective in nociceptive pain but less effective in neuropathic pain (Rang et al. 2016). As well as having analgesic proprieties due to being agonists of opioid receptors, morphine also reduces the affective component of pain, altering the perception of pain (Rang et al. 2016; Waller et al. 2014). Because of the lack of selectivity of opioids, they display a range of side effects, including respiratory depression, euphoria and constipation. It should be noted that there can be significant inter-patient variability in patients' sensitivity to opioid analgesics, due to altered drug metabolism or sensitivity of receptors (Rang et al. 2016). Patients can also develop tolerance and dependence, which is a major concern with prescribing of this class of drug. A public health campaign called *Opioids Aware* has been started by the Royal College of Anaesthetists' Faculty of Pain Medicine in partnership with Public Health England. For links to the resources available as part of this, see the further reading at the end of the chapter (Faculty of Pain Medicine 2016).

Antidepressants: Tricyclic antidepressants such as amitriptyline are commonly used to treat neuropathic pain. They act centrally by inhibiting noradrenaline uptake. They work independently of their antidepressant action and are initiated at doses much lower than the doses that would be used for treating depression. Duloxetine and venlafaxine are also effective. They also inhibit noradrenaline uptake but, in addition, inhibit serotonin uptake. The selective serotonin reuptake inhibitors (SSRIs) are not effective for this indication.

Antiepileptics: Gabapentin and pregabalin are effective in treating neuropathic pain. They act centrally to increase the neurotransmitter GABA, which is involved in stabilising neural tissue. They are particularly effective in treating pain associated with nerve damage (Rang et al. 2016). Both of these drugs have the potential to be misused, and in 2014 PHE and NHS England jointly published advice to support prescribers to prescribe these drugs safely. In 2018, it was announced that due to the continuing concerns about drug misuse, they would be reclassified as Class C controlled substances (Home Office 2018). Carbamazepine is an antiepileptic that acts to stabilise membranes by blocking voltage-gated sodium channels. It only appears to be effective in the treatment of trigeminal neuralgia and is not recommended for treating any other type of pain.

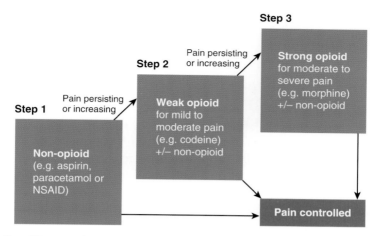

Figure 6.6 – The analgesic ladder

Source: Based on WHO's cancer pain ladder for adults. Available: https://www.who.int/cancer/palliative/painladder/en/.

The Analgesic Ladder

A stepwise approach to managing pain was developed by the World Health Organization (WHO) in 1986. It advocates that analgesia is increased through three steps:

Step 1: Non-opioid analgesics such as paracetamol and NSAIDs should be used.

Step 2: Opioids suitable for mild to moderate pain should be used (+/- non-opioid).

Step 3: Opioids suitable for moderate to severe pain should be used (+/- non-opioid).

This approach can be thought of as a 'step-ladder' and was developed to improve the pain management in patients with cancer pain due to a reluctance to use opioids. The principles have since been applied to acute pain management. For example, severe pain is usually managed straight away with strong opioids and then reduced in a stepwise approach as pain resolves. There is, however, a recognition that it has limitations, as it has never been validated in non-cancer chronic pain (NICE 2017). Increasing the strength of medication also does not take into account the complexity of prescribing for a condition that is influenced by other factors, such as psychological needs and patient priorities.

Chronic Pain Management

Chronic pain management should support patients in dealing with both the physical and psychological elements of their pain. It is unlikely that any pharmacological treatment will completely eliminate chronic pain, so the aim of treatment is to reduce pain and improve quality of life. There is evidence that non-pharmacological interventions can also support a reduction in symptoms (NICE 2017). This means that treatment should be patient-centred and pharmacological options should be considered alongside non-pharmacological interventions.

Patients with chronic pain can benefit from medicines optimisation and shared decision making (NICE 2017). Turn to **Chapter 11** for more on these topics.

Key Points of This Chapter

♦ Therapeutics often involves a stepwise approach to treating patients, with treatment intensified if therapeutic targets are not met.

♦ Regular monitoring and review are crucial to optimise therapeutic outcomes.

♦ Patients with COPD, chronic heart failure and diabetes can all benefit from non-pharmacological interventions and these form a vital part of the therapeutic management.

♦ The inhaler technique is crucial to optimising treatment in COPD. Most patients can learn to use inhalers but they need education and follow-up.

♦ Using the minimum different type of inhaler helps patients get the most out of their treatment.

♦ Antimicrobial stewardship is essential if resistance to antibiotics is to be addressed.

♦ Treatment for pain that is nociceptive or neuropathic in origin varies due to the different pathology of the pain.

Conclusion

It is a complex issue to achieve optimal therapeutic outcomes in patients in practice, particularly for those with long-term conditions. It involves a balancing act between an understanding of the pathophysiology of the disease and of the pharmacology of the drugs used, and patient factors such as any other co-morbidities and their willingness or ability to engage with treatment.

It helps to have the following:

♦ Engagement with patients from the very beginning to ensure that the patient is happy with and is realistically able to manage whatever decisions are made

♦ Clear therapeutic goals

♦ A plan for appropriate monitoring and review of treatment
♦ Working as part of an MDT, e.g. with HF or diabetes specialist teams and clear communication between members of the team.

References and Further Reading

British National Formulary (BNF) *British Medical Association and Royal Pharmaceutical Society of Great Britain*. London: BNF. (Regular updates are published every quarter – make sure you use the most up-to-date edition or use the online version available on the NICE website.)

SPCs for all the medicines in this chapter can be found at EMC Medicines: https://www.medicines.org.uk/emc.

COPD

Brennan, K. (ed.) (2019) NICE Bites 115: Chronic obstructive pulmonary disease. North West Medicines Information Centre. Available at: https://www.sps.nhs.uk/articles/nice-bites-copd.

Magnussen, H., Disse, B., Rodriguez-Roisin, R. et al. (2014) Withdrawal of inhaled glucocorticoids and exacerbations of COPD. *New England Journal of Medicine* 371(14): 1285–1294.

Mak, V. (2017) Treatment guidelines for COPD – going for GOLD? *Primary Care Respiratory Update* 4(2): 19–24.

National Institute for Clinical Excellence (NICE) (2018a) Chronic obstructive pulmonary disease in over 16s: Diagnosis and management [NG115]. Available at: https://www.nice.org.uk/guidance/ng115.

National Institute for Clinical Excellence (NICE) (2018b) Stop smoking interventions and services [NG92]. Available at: https://www.nice.org.uk/guidance/ng92

National Institute for Clinical Excellence (NICE) (2019) NICE clinical knowledge summary: Chronic obstructive pulmonary disease. Available at: https://cks.nice.org.uk/chronic-obstructive-pulmonary-disease#!scenario.

Pearce, L. (2011) How to teach inhaler technique. *Nursing Times* 107(8): 16–17.

Pearce, L. (2012) Responsible prescribing for asthma and COPD. *Nursing Times* 108(46): 12–16.

Rang, H. P., Ritter, J.M., Flower, R. J. et al. (2015) *Rang and Dale's Pharmacology*. London: Elsevier.

Walker, R. and Whittlesea, C. (eds) (2018) *Clinical Pharmacy and Therapeutics*. Oxford: Elsevier/Churchill Livingstone, Chapter 26, pp. 457–474.

Wan, Y. (2013) Is there any evidence to support the use of enteric coated (EC) over uncoated prednisolone tablets? Available at: https://www.sps.nhs.uk/articles/is-there-any-evidence-to-support-the-use-of-enteric-coated-ec-over-uncoated-prednisolone-tablets/ (last accessed: 27 January 2020).

Chronic Heart Failure

British National Formulary (BNF), British Medical Association (BMA) and the Royal Pharmaceutical Society (RPS) (2019a) Angiotensin-Converting Enzyme Inhibitors.

Available at: https://bnf.nice.org.uk/drug-class/angiotensin-converting-enzyme-inhibitors.html#monitoringRequirements.

British National Formulary (BNF), British Medical Association (BMA) and the Royal Pharmaceutical Society (RPS) (2019b) Treatment summary for chronic heart failure. Available at: https://bnf.nice.org.uk/treatment-summary/chronic-heart-failure.html.

National Institute for Clinical Excellence (NICE) (2018) Chronic heart failure in adults: diagnosis and management [NG 106]. Available at: https://www.nice.org.uk/guidance/ng106.

Neal, M. (2016) *Medical Pharmacology at a Glance*. Oxford: Wiley-Blackwell.

Ponikowski, P., Voors, A. A., Anker, S. D. et al. (2016) 2016 ESC Guidelines for the diagnosis and treatment of acute and chronic heart failure. The Task Force for the diagnosis and treatment of acute and chronic heart failure of the European Society of Cardiology (ESC). *European Heart Journal* 37: 2129–2200.

Pitt, B. Ferreira, J. P and Zannad, F. (2017) Mineralocorticoid receptor antagonists in patients with heart failure: current experience and future perspectives *European Heart Journal – Cardiovascular Pharmacotherapy* 3: 1, 48–57.

Rang, H. P., Ritter, J. M., Flower, R. J. et al. (2016) *Rang and Dale's Pharmacology*. London: Elsevier.

Scottish Intercollegiate Guideline Network (SIGN) (2016) SIGN 147: Treatment of chronic heart failure. Available at: https://www.sign.ac.uk/assets/sign147.pdf.

South West London Medicines Optimisation Group (2017) Pharmacological management of chronic heart failure. Available at: http://www.swlmcg.nhs.uk/Clinical/Cardiovascular/HEART%20FAILURE%20-%20Pharmacological%20Management%20of%20Heart%20Failure.pdf.

Walker, R. and Whittlesea, C. (eds) (2018) *Clinical Pharmacy and Therapeutics*. Oxford: Elsevier/Churchill Livingstone, Chapter 21.

Waller, D., Sampson, A., Renwick, A. et al. (2014) *Medical Pharmacology and Therapeutics*. London: Saunders Elsevier.

Diabetes Mellitus

Medicines and Healthcare products Regulatory Authority (MHRA) (2011) Pioglitazone: risk of bladder cancer. Available at: https://www.gov.uk/drug-safety-update/pioglitazone-risk-of-bladder-cancer.

Medicines and Healthcare products Regulatory Authority (MHRA) (2016) SGLT2 inhibitors: Updated advice on the risk of diabetic ketoacidosis. Available at: https://www.gov.uk/drug-safety-update/sglt2-inhibitors-updated-advice-on-the-risk-of-diabetic-ketoacidosis (last accessed 26 February 2020).

National Institute for Clinical Excellence (NICE) (2008). Continuous subcutaneous insulin infusion for the treatment of diabetes mellitus [TA151]. Available at: https://www.nice.org.uk/guidance/ta151.

National Institute for Clinical Excellence (NICE) (2015a) Type 2 diabetes in adults: Management NICE guideline [NG28]. Available at: https://www.nice.org.uk/guidance/ng28.

National Institute for Clinical Excellence (NICE) (2016) NICE clinical knowledge summary: Type 1 diabetes. Available at: https://cks.nice.org.uk/diabetes-type-1.

National Institute for Clinical Excellence (NICE) (2019) NICE clinical knowledge summary: Type 2 diabetes. Available at: https://cks.nice.org.uk/diabetes-type-2.

Neal, M. (2016) *Medical Pharmacology at a Glance*. Oxford: Wiley-Blackwell.

Rang, H. P., Ritter, J. M., Flower, R. J. et al. (2015) *Rang and Dale's Pharmacology*. London: Elsevier.

Walker, R. and Whittlesea, C. (eds) (2018) *Clinical Pharmacy and Therapeutics*. Oxford: Elsevier/Churchill Livingstone.

Waller, D., Sampson, A., Renwick, A. et al. (2014) *Medical Pharmacology and Therapeutics*. London: Saunders Elsevier.

Managing Infections

National Institute for Clinical Excellence (NICE) (2015b) Antimicrobial stewardship: Systems and processes for effective antimicrobial medicine use [NG15]. London: NICE. Available at: https://www.nice.org.uk/guidance/NG15/chapter/1-Recommendations#all-antimicrobials.

National Institute for Clinical Excellence (NICE) (2016) Antimicrobial stewardship quality standard [QS121]. London: NICE. Available at: https://www.nice.org.uk/guidance/qs121.

National Institute for Clinical Excellence (NICE) (2018) Urinary tract infection (lower): antimicrobial prescribing. London: NICE. Available at: https://www.nice.org.uk/guidance/ng109/resources/visual-summary-pdf-6544021069.

Neal, M. (2016) *Medical Pharmacology at a Glance*. Oxford: Wiley-Blackwell.

Rang, H. P., Ritter, J. M., Flower, R. J. et al. (2015) *Rang and Dale's Pharmacology*. London: Elsevier.

Royal College of General Practitioners (RCGP) (n.d.) Target toolkit. Available at: https://www.rcgp.org.uk/targetantibiotics.

Walker, R. and Whittlesea, C. (eds) (2018) *Clinical Pharmacy and Therapeutics*. Oxford: Elsevier/Churchill Livingstone.

World Health Organization (WHO) (2018) Antibiotic resistance. Available at: https://www.who.int/news-room/fact-sheets/detail/antibiotic-resistance.

Managing Pain

British Pain Society (BPS) (2013) *Guidelines for Pain Management Programmes for Adults*. London: BPS.

Faculty of Pain Medicine (2016) Opioids aware: A resource for patients and healthcare professionals to support prescribing of opioid medicines for pain. London: Royal College of Anaesthetists. Available at: http://www.fpm.ac.uk/faculty-of-pain-medicine/opioids-aware.

Home Office (2018) Pregabalin and gabapentin to be controlled as Class C drugs. Available at: https://www.gov.uk/government/news/pregabalin-and-gabapentin-to-be-controlled-as-class-c-drugs.

National Institute for Clinical Excellence (NICE) (2015c) Clinical knowledge summary: Analgesia – mild to moderate pain. London: NICE. Available at: https://cks.nice.org.uk/analgesia-mild-to-moderate-pain.

National Institute for Clinical Excellence (NICE) (2017) Medicines optimisation in chronic pain: Key therapeutic topic [KTT21]. London: NICE. Available at: https://www.nice.org.uk/advice/ktt21/chapter/Evidence-context#managing-chronic-pain.

Neal, M. (2016) *Medical Pharmacology at a Glance*. Oxford: Wiley-Blackwell.

NHS Choices (n.d.) 10 ways to reduce pain. Available at: https://www.nhs.uk/live-well/healthy-body/10-ways-to-ease-pain/.

Public Health England (PHE) and NHS England (2014) Pregabalin and gabapentin: Advice for prescribers on the risk of misuse. Available at: https://www.gov.uk/government/publications/pregabalin-and-gabapentin-advice-for-prescribers-on-the-risk-of-misuse.

Rang, H. P., Ritter, J. M., Flower, R. J. et al. (2016) *Rang and Dale's Pharmacology*. London: Elsevier.

Royal College of Nursing (RCN) (n.d.) Subject guide: Pain. Updated 2019. Available at: https://www.rcn.org.uk/library/subject-guides/pain.

Walker, R. and Whittlesea, C. (eds) (2018) *Clinical Pharmacy and Therapeutics*. Oxford: Elsevier/Churchill Livingstone.

Chapter 7
Evidence-based Medicine

Jennifer Gorman

In This Chapter

- ♦ Introduction
- ♦ Background to evidence-based medicine
- ♦ Local and national approaches to evidence-based prescribing
- ♦ Monitoring prescribing costs
- ♦ Assessing the 'value' of medicines
- ♦ Measuring and comparing health outcomes
- ♦ What are the different types of evidence and when are they useful?
- ♦ How to review and interpret evidence
- ♦ Key points of this chapter
- ♦ Conclusion
- ♦ References and further reading.

Introduction

As a prescriber, you will constantly be having to make clinical decisions about the treatments you prescribe for patients. There is such a wealth of evidence available that it can be difficult to make sense of how this applies to individual prescribing practice. The aim of this chapter is not to try and turn you into a health economist or master statistician, but to support you practically in understanding and using evidence to inform your clinical decisions. We will start by looking at how evidence-based medicine is used to inform some of the prescribing support you will be accessing at both a local and a national level through formularies and guidelines. We will also consider the costs of medicines and how these costs are monitored. Cost is only one element of a decision to prescribe and so we will explore how the 'value' of a medicine can be quantified in terms of health outcomes and the concept of cost-effective prescribing. We will look at what types of evidence there are and some of their pros and cons. In the final part of the chapter we will look at developing your skills in taking a piece of evidence, reviewing it and then applying it to your practice.

Background to Evidence-based Medicine

In an article in the BMJ entitled 'Evidence-based medicine: what it is and what it isn't', evidence-based medicine was described as 'the conscientious, explicit, and judicious use of current best evidence in making decisions about the care of individual patients' (Sackett et al. 1996, p. 71).

How it has been interpreted and applied in practice varies and there are those who believe this approach has a negative impact on patient care by restricting clinical judgement. However, this definition does acknowledge that a key factor is clinical expertise. The skill comes in being able to integrate the evidence and your expertise in making decisions about your patients.

Local and National Approaches to Evidence-based Prescribing

Historically, clinicians employed an empirical approach to their medical practice. They tried out treatments on their patients and if they observed that they worked, then they would use them in other similar cases. Clinicians would build up a preferred range of treatments for their patients based on clinical experience. The introduction of the licensing of medicines means that there is now a standardised approach to the process of testing medicines. This ensures that both the efficacy and safety of individual medicines is independently verified. The clinical trials used in testing medicines, however, only give us information about one specific drug and often only compare the drug to a placebo. In an effort to reduce variation and improve the quality of prescribing, there has been a widespread acceptance of the use of clinical guidelines and formularies. These are developed to support evidence-based prescribing.

Local Prescribing and Evidence-based Medicine

The NHS Constitution for England was first published in 2009, and one of the things it was designed to address was variation in local decision making, leading to variations in access to medicines (NPC 2009). Various guidance documents were developed to support the production of local formularies, where the use of medicines was based on both evidence and the needs of the local population, with a view to improving both the quality and cost-effectiveness of prescribing.

Since then, NICE has produced guidance that supports the development of local formularies (NICE 2014a). It has defined a local formulary as 'the output of processes to support the managed introduction, utilisation or withdrawal of healthcare treatments within a local health economy' (NICE 2014a). The output produced is essentially a list of medicines, which have been considered by a local decision-making body such as Area Prescribing Committees (APCs), which supports a rational approach to prescribing. Local formularies may tell us when medicines shouldn't be prescribed or give a first-line preference in a drug class; for example, they may tell us which one is first-line if statin therapy is needed.

In current clinical practice, Clinical Commissioning Groups (CCGs) are responsible for overseeing the production of local formularies and guidelines that support their prescribers in making evidence-based decisions. As part of the formulary development process, the evidence about the safety, efficacy and cost-effectiveness of the drug is taken into account. These are agreed by the APC, which are collaborative committees with representatives from different care settings participating in decision making. This means that there should be a joint approach to the formulary across both primary and secondary care.

Drugs that are included on the formulary are placed in different categories which indicate where and by whom the drug is best prescribed. The definitions and categories may vary between localities, so make sure you are familiar with your local area.

Examples of Different Drug Categories You May See on Formularies

Non-formulary: These are drugs that should not routinely be prescribed if there is a formulary choice available, as the evidence for their use has not been appraised and their place in therapy is therefore undetermined. There will be an application process locally for non-formulary drugs to be considered for inclusion on the formulary.

Blacklisted: This means that the evidence for the drug has been appraised by the APC and it has been decided that the drug is not appropriate to use in any care setting.

Drugs that require shared care agreements: These drugs should be prescribed initially in a specialist care setting but, once the patient is stable, prescribing can be taken over in general practice. There are criteria in the agreement that outline what responsibility both parties take in the ongoing care of the patient.

Red drugs: Drugs that are coded as red have been assessed by as only being suitable for prescribing in a specialist setting.

You may wonder why we need local formularies – why not just have one large national formulary? It is a good question, especially in response to the concept of the postcode lottery of healthcare. The flexibility that local formularies give local areas means they can prioritise how they spend their allocated budget for their specific population based on factors such as demography or geography. This means the local needs of patients can be prioritised, and by making sure the formulary supports the cost-effective use of medicines, more patients can receive treatment. This is certainly not purely about cost saving, but about improving access to medicines and improving the quality of care patients receive. It involves reducing clinical risk by ensuring that medicines can be used safely and in an appropriate care setting, which may vary between localities depending on how services are commissioned. It also involves thinking about optimising patient outcomes, in terms of both mortality and morbidity in the patient population in the local area.

Summary of Some of the Potential Benefits of Local Formularies:
- ◆ Improve the quality of local care pathways that include medicines and prescribing
- ◆ Improve the quality of prescribing through improved access to medicines and reduction in variation of clinical care
- ◆ Encourage a joint approach to prescribing across the health economy. This can support a joined-up approach to supply arrangements, as well as financial management across the health community.

Think about:

- ◆ Do you know how to access the most up-to-date version of your local formulary? (Check the internet to find the online version if you don't usually access it this way.)
- ◆ Do you know any drugs that are prescribed under shared care in your local area? Is there anything you would need to consider if you were prescribing for that patient in terms of extra information to the GP?
- ◆ What reasons do you think there may be for APCs deciding a drug should not be prescribed locally?

Clinical Guidelines

Clinical guidelines are designed to support clinicians and patients making choices about care based on a systematic approach to the evidence available. In practice it is impossible to keep up to date and assimilate all the evidence that is constantly being published in healthcare. This evidence can include things like changes in the criteria for diagnosing a condition, criteria for referral or the best treatment options. The purpose of clinical guidelines is to do that work for you by producing statements based on systematic review of the evidence that include recommendations to support best clinical practice and improve patient care (Graham et al. 2011). It is important to consider which guidelines you use, as unfortunately not all guidance is created equally. There should be a rigorous and transparent development process. There should be consideration given to who is involved in the development process, how evidence is identified and appraised, how the guideline is put together and what the review process is. It should produce guidelines that are based on the best available evidence and provide support that is clinically applicable and easy to use in practice. There should be a schedule for review based on the likelihood that the evidence contained in the guideline will become outdated. For more information on the process that NICE uses to develop its guidelines, see its guidelines manual (NICE 2014b).

NICE is the most well-known organisation which produces national clinical guidelines in the UK. It makes evidence-based recommendations on a wide range of topics from preventing and managing specific conditions, to providing social care and planning broader services and interventions to improve health (NICE 2014b).

It is important to be aware of the range of information that NICE produces and what impact it can have on prescribing. The three most relevant areas are technology appraisals, clinical guidelines and quality standards. These are outlined below.

Technology appraisal (TA): When a positive TA is published by NICE, the NHS has a statutory requirement to provide funding within 30–90 days of publication. TAs can look at a range of medical interventions, and medicines are one of these. For example, New Oral Anti-Coagulants (NOACs) are a class of medicines that have TAs associated with their use. This means that the NHS must follow what is contained within these TAs in terms of the treatments it offers to patients. (Please note that the TA refers to NOACs, but since its publication the term DOAC has come into use for the same group of drugs.)

Clinical guidance (NG): Unlike a TA, the NHS is not obliged to implement the recommendations in an NG. However, a clinical guideline, like a TA, is developed looking at the clinical efficacy and the economic impact of a drug or treatment pathway. This means that ideally these would be followed. There may, however, be occasions when this does not happen in practice. One reason is that the infrastructure is not in place to support prescribers to follow the guidance. Another is that the guideline may become outdated. One example of this is in COPD treatment. NICE published guidance in 2010 on diagnosing and managing COPD, but this was not updated until 2018. During this time, treatment moved on and many prescribers looked for guidelines that provided more up-to-date information (Mak 2017). One such guideline is produced by the GOLD (Global Initiative for Chronic Obstructive Lung Disease) global strategy for diagnosis, management and prevention of COPD. It was found in a survey of the Primary Care Respiratory Society in 2017 that 65% of respondents were following GOLD guidance and only 33% NICE guidance (Mak 2017). If you prescribe for a patient, and are not following an NG, then it is important to have a clear rationale for your decision.

Quality standards (QS): These standards are designed to help improve the quality of care that is being provided or commissioned. They define what high-quality care should look like and allow comparisons to be made with current practice. NICE says that they can be used to:

♦ Identify gaps and areas for improvement
♦ Measure quality of care
♦ Understand how to improve care
♦ Demonstrate you provide quality care
♦ Commission high-quality services.

There are a range of case studies on the NICE website that illustrate how quality standards have been used in practice to improve patient care (available at: https://www.nice.org.uk/standards-and-indicators/how-to-use-quality-standards).

Monitoring Prescribing Costs

As we have already seen, the economic impact of a drug is a significant factor in prescribing decisions. This is not surprising, as the King's Fund (Ewbank et al. 2018) found that the cost of medicines to the NHS rose from £13 billion in 2010/2011 to £17.4 billion in 2016/2017. This pattern of increasing costs is unlikely to change, as there are more patients requiring medicines. Also, as drugs become more sophisticated, the cost of new medicines coming on to the market is increasing.

What this means is that there are a whole range of competing factors that policy-makers, commissioners and individual prescribers have to take into account when providing care for patients. It also means that data about prescribing from the CCG level down to individual prescribers is collected and monitored. Whilst financial management is important, monitoring prescribing is not just about saving money on the prescribing budget; it is also about driving up quality and improving practice and thinking about the costs to the wider health economy. For example, if COPD patients are well managed, their treatment is optimised and exacerbations will be reduced. This high-quality prescribing means that overall the cost to the health economy will be reduced, as money will be saved by not having to manage the exacerbations. It can also reduce the potential of patients suffering from adverse effects. For example, if it is noticed that patients in a local area being treated for asthma are on unusually high doses of steroids, then work can be done to support them in stepping down treatment. This can result in a saving on the cost of inhaled therapy, but also reduces the risk of long-term side effects that will need managing at a later date.

How Monitoring Prescribing Can Improve Quality

♦ Highlighting inappropriate and unsafe practice
♦ Reducing waste
♦ Ensuring patients have access to the most appropriate treatments.

Prescribing Data

All prescriptions that are dispensed against are processed by the NHS Prescription Authority, part of the NHS Business Services Authority (NHSBSA). This is ostensibly so that pharmacies can claim payment for the medicines they have supplied, and thus only includes prescriptions actually dispensed. This data is also released quarterly by the NHSBSA, meaning that CCGs can access data on prescribing from all prescribers associated with a GP practice, whether that be GPs or other independent prescribers. The resulting data is known as ePACT (electronic prescribing analysis and costing) data and it can be interrogated to provide a range of cost-based analyses. For more detailed information on practice level data, see the NHS digital website: https://digital. nhs.uk/data-and-information/areas-of-interest/prescribing.

Access to ePACT data is managed by CCGs, but you can access NHSBSA prescribing data using the OpenPrescribing website (available at: https:// openprescribing.net). This is free to use by anyone and you can download prescribing data to GP practice level. There is a useful FAQ section that guides you through how to use the site and interpret the data.

Think about:

♦ How does your practice access ePACT data?
♦ What do they use it for?
♦ How will this impact your prescribing practice?

Assessing the 'Value' of Medicines

How do we assess what 'value' a medicine has? We have talked about how funds are limited, and medicines are assessed nationally and locally to determine their place in therapy. Included in this assessment is the difficult reality of how economic factors influence prescribing. However, the 'value' of a medicine goes beyond only its cost; a medicine is potentially something that can save a life or relieve suffering. It can also actually have a positive economic impact by keeping someone in work to contribute financially to society through taxes. Weighing these things up can help us to ascribe a nominal 'value' to a medicine. In health economics value is often measured by quantitatively relating cost to health outcomes (Moore and McQuay 2006). There are various terms and measures that are used, some of which will be discussed now. This is only a brief overview of this subject; if you want to find out more, explore some of the references given at the end of the chapter.

Cost-effectiveness

Cost-effectiveness measures drug costs against health outcomes. It is about balancing what represents value for money for the NHS with what is effective for the patient, by comparing the health gains of interventions against their monetary cost. We can have a drug that is very cheap, but if it is prescribed for a large number of patients, then the cost to the NHS as a whole can become significant. However, if the evidence shows that the drug reduces mortality and morbidity in these patients, then prescribing it can be viewed as cost-effective. If the effect on mortality and morbidity is negligible across the patient group as a whole, then we could take a different view.

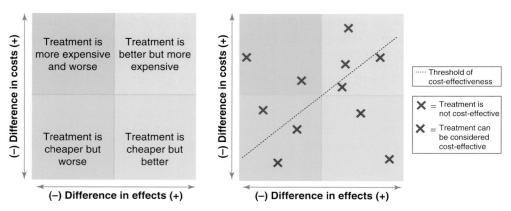

Figure 7.1 – The cost-effectiveness plane

This can be represented visually using the cost-effectiveness plane shown in Figure 7.1.

What this illustrates is that decisions about whether a drug is cost-effective are made based on not only the cost, but also the difference in the effect produced in patients compared with other treatments. It shows that even if a new drug is more expensive, it may still be accepted for use in practice if it is able to produce enough of an effect on patient outcomes. The line through the middle of the plane is the threshold below which the drug can be considered as acceptable for use. These thresholds are necessary in a health system that does not have finite funds. They also protect patients from being exposed to treatments that do not provide a significant enough health benefit.

Let's use the example of statins to think about cost-effectiveness. NICE guidelines on lipid modification recommend statins as primary prevention for cardiovascular disease (CVD) in the following situations:

♦ In those patients with a QRISK score of more than 10%
♦ Patients who have type 1 diabetes, chronic kidney disease or familial hypercholesterolaemia
♦ Patients who are over 85 years old should be considered for therapy without the need for a formal risk assessment based on the risk versus benefit of treatment and other co-morbidities.

Thinking about the patients you see in practice, you will appreciate there is a large cohort of patients eligible for treatment under these criteria. Although the cost of these drugs is minimal compared to the cost of, for example, many cancer therapies, the number of patients on treatment will be much larger. This is why NICE has specified specific clinical parameters, such as the QRISK score, because in these patients the reduction seen in CVD is calculated to be cost-effective. This is because CVD itself has associated costs, from societal costs and lost workdays to the treatments the patients who develop CVD will subsequently need. This means, essentially, that the cost of the drug can be evaluated against the cost saved through the number cases of CVD prevented. This can tell us if it is cost-effective to prescribe. This only holds for the group of patients the evaluation takes place in; if the group of patients changes, then the cost-effectiveness analysis could change.

So, some questions we might be interested in when considering cost-effectiveness are:

♦ What is the price of the drug itself to the NHS?
♦ What are any associated peripheral costs, e.g. monitoring or administering?
♦ What outcome will this have for the patient and can we quantify any costs associated with this, e.g. ability to work?
♦ What patient group is this relevant to?
♦ If a drug is not cost-effective in the whole patient group, can we define a specific population in the patient group in which it will be cost-effective? (E.g. a drug may not be cost-effective to be prescribed for all diabetic patients, but it may become so in diabetic patients who have a certain level of chronic kidney disease (CKD)).

Think about:

Imagine you have to decide whether a new treatment for a diabetes drug is cost-effective. It is a drug that has been licensed to improve glycaemic control. What are the key questions you would want to know the answer to before you made a decision?

Answers:

♦ What type of diabetes is it licensed for (this can affect the population size and the method of administration and potentially the number of years that treatment will be needed)?
♦ What is the net cost of the drug?
♦ What is the cost of any equipment needed to administer (e.g. if it is injectable)?
♦ What evidence is there to demonstrate that the drug improves glycaemic control or other clinical outcomes?
♦ Can the impact on the quantity and quality of life for the patient be quantified?
♦ What place in therapy will it have (e.g. will patients all start on it at diagnosis or will it be something they only have if other treatments aren't working)?

Case Study 7.1

You have an appointment with Mrs Jones in her home. She is a 59-year-old patient who you last saw two days ago. Your diagnosis was Eron Class 1 mild cellulitis and you initiated the patient on flucloxacillin 500 grams QDS as per local antimicrobial guidelines. You have returned to review the patient and at the review you find that the cellulitis has spread beyond the area you marked on your last visit. You perform a full clinical assessment and now assess her cellulitis as Eron Class 2 moderate cellulitis. This means that IV treatment is indicated according to local antimicrobial guidelines. She does, however, remain ambulatory and has support at home from her husband who is fit and well.

Historically, this would have automatically meant that the patient would need to be admitted to hospital for treatment. Many local areas have, however, developed outpatient parenteral antibiotic therapy (OPAT) pathways where patients can receive IV antibiotics in their home for this condition. If you are not familiar with the details of these pathways, see the references at the end of the chapter for further reading.

Activity: List any factors linked to either patient outcomes or cost that you think influenced why and how these pathways were developed. Include any factors that might influence the choice of antibiotics used as part of these pathways:

♦ It can prevent an acute admission for something that evidence supports can safely be managed at home. Acute admissions are extremely expensive relative to at-home care. It also reduces the risk to the patient of hospital-acquired infections.

♦ Although the pathway should deliver overall cost savings by reducing bed days in hospital, there is a cost implication to providing the treatment in a different care setting. The funding of this would need to have been factored into the cost analysis by commissioners when designing the service.

♦ Antibiotics used in inpatient treatment may not be suitable for use in primary care due to the practicalities of administration – for example, an infusion given over a long period or a drug that has to be given multiple times per day would not be suitable in the community. Flucloxacillin is not used for this reason, as it requires four times daily administration. Commonly used antibiotics are teicoplanin and ceftriaxone, both of which are once daily.

♦ One final consideration to ensure that both patient outcomes and cost-effectiveness are optimised is to ensure that the IV to oral switch takes place at the appropriate time.

Measuring and Comparing Health Outcomes

We have talked already about comparing interventions based on cost and the health gains they provide. In this section, we will think in more detail about how these health gains are measured to allow this comparison to take place.

For some drugs this may seem relatively simple, as there is a specific measurement or objective assessment that can take place. Let's go back to the example of statins. In clinical trials on statins, data may be collected on specific biological measurements, such as serum cholesterol and triglycerides. In this way, the change within the body produced by the drug can be measured. This is great, but does not actually tell us how many people will be saved from having a myocardial infarction (MI) or a stroke if they take these drugs. The data needs to be related to a measure that can help us decide if the health outcome the drug provides is actually worth us prescribing it. The NICE (2014c) patient decision aid on lipid modification provides this is the kind of information. It shows the different reductions in morbidity linked to the different QRISK scores in patients taking statins at therapeutic doses.

So, as **Figure 7.2** shows, if a patient with a QRISK of 10% takes a statin for the next ten years, they have 4% less chance of developing coronary heart disease (CHD) or stroke.

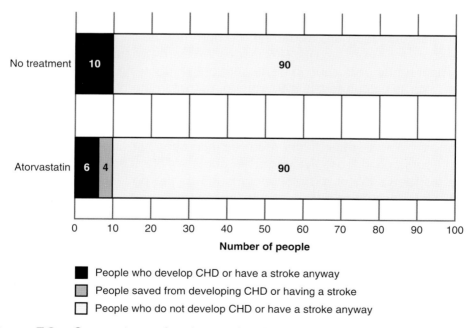

Figure 7.2 – Comparison of patients who develop CHD or stroke over ten years with atorvastatin versus no treatment in patients with a 10% QRISK
Source: NICE (2014c).

For more information on using patient decision aids in shared decision making, turn to **Chapter 11**.

This gives us a figure that can help a patient decide in balancing their own perception of risk and benefit of a particular treatment. However, it gives us no information on how the statin will affect the quality or quantity of the patient's life. In reality, treatments are related to health outcomes that are more complex than binary 'does it happen?' or 'does it not happen?' questions. It is therefore useful to be able to have an estimate of how both quantity and quality of life are impacted during treatment.

This means that more complex ways of relating cost and health outcomes are needed and it is these that are often used by policy-makers and commissioners. These are known as quality indices, and one which is commonly used that you may have come across is the QALY (quality-adjusted life year).

Case Study 7.2

Imagine one of your patients, Mr Khan, has cancer. He is prescribed a chemotherapy drug that will extend his life expectancy by two years. The side effects of this treatment are horrendous, and so his quality of life score falls from 1 to 0.3. This means the extra two years that he gains is offset by the reduction in his quality of life following treatment. When the QALY is calculated, it is 0.6, meaning that in the two years extra he will only gain 0.6 years in perfect health.

Imagine now Mrs Cowling, who is one of your patients being treated for diabetes. The treatment she receives increases her life expectancy by five years and in those five years her quality of life score falls to 0.7. This means the QALY for this treatment is 3.5 as the patient can expect an extra 3.5 years in perfect health following treatment.

These figures are relatively crude and should be taken in context, but they do allow some way of rationalising decisions on medicines. NICE currently has a cost-effectiveness threshold of £20,000–£30,000 per QALY, with drugs having a cost above this not usually being recommended. This means that if the cost of the cancer treatment in the example above was £25,000, it is less likely to be recommended as the QALY is only 0.6. Conversely if the diabetes treatment cost the same amount, it is more likely to be considered as the QALY is 3.5.

Definition of a QALY: This is a measure that relates quality of life to quantity of life. It is calculated estimating the years of life remaining for a patient following a particular treatment or intervention and weighting each year with a quality-of-life score (on a 0 to 1 scale) (definition from NICE: https://www.nice.org.uk/glossary). One QALY is equal to one year of life in perfect health. If a treatment extends a patient's life by one year but they do not have perfect health, maybe suffering from pain or fatigue, then this is taken into account and the QALY will be less than 1.

What are the Different Types of Evidence and When are They Useful?

So far, we have focused on decision making mostly in the context of how guidance and support is developed by policy-makers and commissioners. We will now focus on the evidence itself, starting with the types of evidence. Most people are familiar with the concept of clinical trials, but these can be run in a multitude of different ways. There are also a range of other types of evidence, from systematic reviews to cohort studies and case reports.

Research can be broadly divided into two types depending on the type of information it provides: quantitative and qualitative.

Quantitative: research that includes an outcome measure that provides numerical data combined with statistical analysis.

Qualitative: this does not quantify the outcomes but evaluates factors such as perception, experience or understanding as a more subjective entity.

Research that focuses on medicines is by its nature normally quantitative as we are looking to objectively define the effect an intervention has on specific parameters. Even research that looks at subjective topics, such as pain management, will aim to be quantitative by measuring changes in pain using validated scoring systems. The advantage of this approach is that it allows comparisons to be made more easily between different treatments.

Attempts have been made to provide guidance for healthcare professionals on what type of research might give us the most robust evidence on which to base our decisions. The Oxford CEBM (2009) published guidelines assigning 'levels' to different types of evidence. Figure 7.3 summarises these levels. The evidence obtained using the methods at the top of the pyramid is deemed to provide more rigorous evidence on which to base decisions. So, ideally all our decisions would be based on systematic reviews and meta-analyses. In practice this evidence may not be available for every drug, so then we would look to randomised controlled trials (RCTs). In some instances, there may not be an RCT for us to go to for evidence, in which case we may need to look to what evidence is available, such as expert opinion. The main thing to remember when considering what type of evidence you should use is whether you have chosen the level of evidence that is most suited to the question you are trying to answer.

The focus in this section will be on the three types of studies at the top of the prescribing pyramid – randomised controlled trials, systematic reviews and meta-analyses. If you want to find out more about other types of quantitative research or qualitative research, use the references at the end of the chapter for further reading.

Randomised Controlled Trials

Randomised controlled trials (RCTs) are types of primary evidence. This means that the researchers actually collect data about patients and it is this data that is evaluated in the results. They are generally considered the 'gold standard' type of primary evidence in assessing the effect of a particular drug intervention. The basic construction of this type of research method is to randomly allocate participants into groups and then give one group the drug under investigation

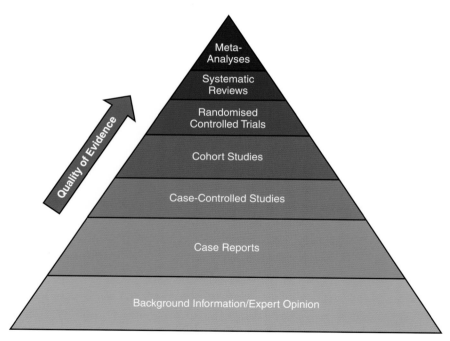

Figure 7.3 – The pyramid of evidence
Source: Adapted from: CFCF / Wikimedia Commons: https://commons.wikimedia.org/wiki/File:Research_design_and_evidence_-_Capho.svg.

with the other group acting as a control. If the trial is designed appropriately, then it should be possible to attribute any change in the outcome measure to the drug rather than to random chance.

Single-blinded RCTs

This type of RCT follows the construction above, but in addition the patients are 'blinded'. This means they do not know whether they have been allocated to the group that is having the intervention or the control group. The researchers conducting the trial are aware of the allocation of patient to either the intervention or the control group. The aim of this is to reduce the risk of bias; for example, if patients know they are receiving a placebo and not an active drug, this may skew the results. It does not however eliminate the risk of bias being introduced, whether intentionally or unintentionally, by the researchers.

Double-blinded RCTs

In this type of RCT neither the patients nor the researchers know which group the patients have been allocated to. The aim of this is to reduce the chance of the results being biased by either group knowing. Because of this, double-blinded RCTs are generally seen as a more rigorous approach. However, they are not always possible depending on the nature of the clinical trial.

Systematic Reviews and Meta-analyses

These are known as secondary evidence. This means that they use more than one source of primary evidence and, by summarising the knowledge in these sources, they can make judgements about what impact this evidence may have on healthcare. A systematic review looks at the research as a whole, whilst meta-analysis focuses on the statistical analysis of the results. Both of these can be extremely complex to do well. There is a specific method that should be used to ensure the results are as representative as possible of the available data, for example to minimise bias when selecting papers to include/exclude. This means that when reading and using these reviews, you should develop your ability to evaluate how well the review has been carried out.

The Cochrane Collection is one of the most well-known organisations that produces high-quality systematic reviews. You can read more about its process at: https://consumers.cochrane.org/what-systematic-review. Other useful resources in helping develop your knowledge about how these reviews are done and how to evaluate them are Greenhalgh (2014) and the CASP checklist on systematic reviews available at: https://casp-uk.net/casp-tools-checklists.

There are many other types of research, but unfortunately we cannot cover them all in this chapter. If you want to find out more about a particular type of research, consider reading Greenhalgh (2014), Moore and McQuay (2006) or Straus et al. (2019).

> **Systematic Review:**
> A systematic review is a structured way of identifying high-quality research on a particular clinical topic and summarising that research. It means that large amounts of information can be synthesised into something that can be used to inform clinical practice.
>
> **Meta-analysis:**
> This focuses on putting together the statistical analysis of different primary research focusing on the same clinical topic. Essentially it allows numerical comparison of different trials through statistical testing. By combining the results, it effectively increases the sample size and there is an increased possibility that we can minimise the risk of chance playing a significant role in the data. This relies on the trials being of good quality and validity.

How to Review and Interpret Evidence

Often much of the work of reviewing and interpreting evidence has been done for us, for example, by NICE when it produces guidance. Unfortunately for those of us who struggle with the thought of statistical analysis, there is no escape from having a basic knowledge of how to read and understand this kind of information about drugs. It may be that you need to be able to answer a question from a patient who asks you about a specific drug and why it is used in preference to another. It may be that a drug company is keen to persuade you that a new drug is much better than one already on the market. Whatever the reason, when reviewing any of the types of evidence described above, you need to be aware of some of the key terminology.

So, you are going to evaluate a clinical trial or systematic review – where do you start?

The Critical Appraisal Skills Programme (CASP) suggests that there are three broad issues that you should have in mind when reviewing evidence:

1. Are the results valid?
2. What are the results?
3. How do they apply to your local practice?

Source: Adapted from CASP Checklists (2018)

Are the Results Valid?

When answering this first question, a good place to start is thinking about what the purpose of the research is and whether it is asking a clear research question. The results are only valid if they answer a valid research question. This means looking at the intervention, the population and the outcome against which the intervention is being measured.

For example, if a systematic review included data from studies on paediatric patients, but actually the research question was based on the efficacy of the intervention in an adult population, then the results would not be valid.

You would also want to consider whether the study design adds validity to the results. In an RCT this means thinking about things like how patients were assigned to different groups, whether there were clear inclusion and exclusion criteria, if patients were accounted for in the final data and if the sample size was large enough.

Inclusion and exclusion criteria help to ensure that the population in the trial is appropriate for the research question.

Inclusion criteria: A list of criteria that patients must meet to be included in the study.

Exclusion criteria: These are criteria that mean patients may be excluded from a trial. For example, in a trial looking at primary prevention of CVD, an exclusion criterion would be if the patient has had a previous MI.

Sample Size and the Power of a Study

Sample size: Why does size matter? It is all to do with chance. If you select a random group of patients and measure the outcome of an intervention, it only gives you information about these patients. You want to be able to have some confidence that your results can be extrapolated to all patients who could benefit from the intervention. Part of this is to do with sample size, and trials should include information on how they determined their sample size to ensure it was large enough.

Example: You include 20 people in a study, and allocate them evenly to receive either the drug under study or a placebo. In the results, would what you observe in those ten patients be exactly what you would expect to see in the 1,000 patients you end up treating? Maybe, but with such a small sample size there is a possibility that what you saw in the study is due to chance.

The power of the study: This relates to the sample and describes the power of the study to detect any variations between the groups being studied.

Example: You can calculate the sample size you would need to give the study a particular level of power to detect any significant differences between the group. It may be that the power level is set at 0.80, meaning that the calculation done to determine the minimum sample size gives an 80% chance that any difference will be detected.

What Are the Results?

If you are confident that the results will be valid based on your review of the study design or review process for a systematic review, then you can move on to looking at the results themselves. Firstly, it is important to think about what it is exactly we are looking for in the results. When reviewing research, you need to ask yourself whether the outcomes measured were clearly defined and how much of an effect the intervention produced in changing the outcomes. There should be a primary outcome defined in the research and, depending on the type of research, possibly secondary outcomes. These will be based on what is known as the null hypothesis.

The Null Hypothesis:

Quantitative hypotheses are predictions that are made about the expected outcomes of relationships between different variables (Creswell and Cresswell 2018). The null hypothesis assumes that there is no relationship between the intervention and the outcome.

Example: A new drug is tested in patients with type 2 diabetes mellitus. The null hypothesis states that there will be no difference in glycaemic control (the primary outcome) between the group given the new drug (the intervention group) and those managed by diet alone (the control group).

This means that the onus is on the research to disprove that there is no difference in glycaemic control between the control and intervention groups.

If the outcomes are clearly defined, then you can move on to considering any difference the results detected between the treatment and the control groups and quantifying how precise the results were through statistical analysis.

So far, we have thought about how to minimise the risk of there being an error in detecting a difference between groups linked to the sample size. The next thing to think about is whether that difference could actually have occurred by chance. This is a concept known as statistical significance, and p-values are used to describe it.

The p-value is a number between 0 and 1. If the p-value is 1, then it is 100% likely that the observed effect happened by chance, so of course the aim is to have a p-value of less than 1. If the p-value is 0, however, then it is impossible that the observed effect in a study happened by chance. As it is almost impossible to be certain that chance did not play a part in the results, in clinical studies a p-value of 0.05 is often used. This means that there is a 1 in 20 possibility that the observed effect happened by chance. In some trials, a more stringent lower p-value of 0.01 or 1 in 100 chance is used. If the p-value is less than the figure of either 0.05 or 0.01, then we can say that the results found are statistically significant. You should remember that statistical significance and clinical significance are not necessarily the same thing. For example, a drug trial can show a statistically significant difference between a parameter measured in the control group and in the treatment group. That doesn't mean that when you use it in your patients they will notice any clinical difference in their condition.

Statistical Significance and P-values:

Imagine you are looking at a set of results and you see that a drug reduced the number of heart attacks in the study group by one more than in the placebo group. How do you know whether that reduction is due to the drug or because of chance?

Research methods should be used that allow us to quantify the risk of it being attributable to chance. The p-value being used in this trial was 0.01.

The researchers report that the p-value is less than 0.01. This means that the reduction in heart attacks found in the trial has less than a 1 in 100 probability of being attributable to chance. So, the result is statistically significant.

If the p-value was greater than 0.01 then the results would not be statistically significant. This is an important concept to understand as it means that although sometimes the results might look great on paper, it still might not be possible to be sure that they are not just due to chance.

The final thing that needs to be considered before looking at the results themselves is how precise the results are. So far, we have considered whether the results could have occurred by chance or not. If we accept that they have not occurred by chance (because the p-value tells us this is the case), then any difference seen in the results between the control and the intervention groups is because of the intervention. What we want to think about now is how precise these results are.

What do we mean by precise? Imagine there is a target and you try and shoot an arrow into its centre. Sometimes you might do it and sometimes you might miss slightly. If you repeat this action 100 times but you only record the results of how close you got to the target ten times, then you might not get a result that precisely matches what happened.

This is what can happen when trials are done, as they are only ever conducted in a sample of a whole population. This means that there can be a lack of precision in the results. We can use statistical analysis to give us an estimation of how far from the mark the results we see are from those we might expect to see if we had results for everyone in the population. This analysis gives us confidence intervals.

Confidence Intervals (CI)

Part of a study design involves setting confidence intervals (CIs). It makes sense that if we are only sampling part of a population, the results obtained may not be 100% precise in showing us the value we would see if we measured the whole population. A confidence interval gives us a range in which we can be confident the true value lies. Normally in drug trials they are set at 95% (though sometimes 90% or 99% may be used). This means that we can be 95% confident that any variation in the figures found from the true value is actually in the range that the interval shows.

Example: A drug is tested in hypertensive patients. The systolic blood pressure readings show a mean decrease from 157 mmHg to 142 mmHg. So the mean reduction in systolic blood pressure is 15 mmHg. A 95% confidence interval gives a range of BP reduction between 12 mmHg and 18 mmHg. This means we can be 95% confident that if we tested everyone with hypertension, the value we would find would be a figure somewhere between 12 and 18mmHg.

You can see from the example above that understanding confidence intervals is essential in interpreting results found in trials. If a trial is concluding that a drug is miraculous as it reduces blood pressure on average by 20% but you see the confidence intervals are extremely wide, you may be cautious in taking this claim at face value. If conversely the confidence interval is very small, then the results are more precise and you can be more confident that the true value is similar to that reported.

The final part of this section looks at some of the commonly used ways results are presented in sources of evidence. The way data can be interpreted statistically is extensive, and so in this section three commonly used statistical measures will be explained: absolute risk reduction (ARR), relative risk reduction (RRR) and number needed to treat (NNT).

To illustrate the different ways statistics are used to present results, an example will be used of an RCT which is run to measure the reduction in risk of having a stroke. The treatment group are given a new drug and the control group a placebo. The following results are found:

	Total participants	Number of participants who did not have a stroke	Number of participants who did have a stroke
Treatment group	100	60	40
Control group	100	40	60

Absolute Risk Reduction

This is the difference in outcomes seen in the control and treatment groups under study.

Firstly, we must calculate the absolute risk for each group, which is the number of events that happened in each group. There are 100 patients in the control group and 60 of them had a stroke, so the absolute risk is 0.6 or 60%. Of the 100 patients in the treatment group, 40 had strokes, so the absolute risk of the treatment group was 0.4 or 40%.

The absolute risk reduction (ARR) is then calculated by taking away the risk of control group from the treatment group:

ARR = ARC (0.6) − ART (0.4)
ARR = 0.2

So, the ARR is 0.2 or, to put it another way, there is a 20% reduction in the risk of having a stroke in the treatment group compared with the control group.

Relative Risk Reduction

The relative risk reduction (RRR) calculates the risk reduction of each group relative to the other.

Firstly, the relative risk is calculated using the absolute risk reduction figures of the treatment and control groups:

RR (relative risk) = ART (0.4) / ARC (0.6)
= 0.66

So, the relative risk of having a stroke in the control group versus the placebo group is 66%.

This can further be quantified into the relative risk reduction:

RRR (relative risk reduction) = (ARC − ART) / ARC
= 0.33

In this study, the relative risk of having a stroke is therefore reduced by 33% in the treatment group compared to the group who received no treatment. This figure is quite different from the ARR of 20% and makes the treatment sound even better. This is why investigators often present the results in terms of RRR in preference to other ways (Straus et al. 2019).

Number Needed to Treat

This figure gives an indication of how many people you would need to treat with an intervention to produce one outcome. If the number needed to treat (NNT) is 1, then that means that everyone you treat will have an outcome. If the NNT is 100, then that means that you have to treat 100 people for one person to have an outcome.

The calculation of NNT shows that in the example above we would need to treat five people to prevent one stroke:

NNT (number needed to treat) = 1 / ARR
NNT = 1/0.2 = 5

There is no ideal NNT as it depends on a range of factors as to what is considered acceptable. If treating an infection with an antibiotic that through sensitivity testing is known to be effective on the strain of bacteria causing the infection, you would hope the NNT would be near to 1. This is because you have already tested the drug on the bacteria and so long as there are no pharmacological factors about the patient that prevent the drug getting to where it needs to go, and it is administered via the correct route, then it should work. Similarly, if you have a patient at the end of their life who needs analgesia, then you would hope that the NNT would be on the low side or else patients will die in pain. If, however, you are looking at long-term prevention over a number of years, e.g. anything linked to a Q-RISK ten-year risk calculation, then a higher NNT would be accepted.

Applying This to Your Local Population

This important final step in assessing evidence means that you apply the results from the study to your practice. It is only through considering a trial as a whole that you are able to think about how the evidence you are reading may apply to your patient population. For example, if you look at a systematic analysis and see that all the studies have inclusion criteria that all patients are children, but you only prescribe for an adult population, then you need look no further at that study. Or, you may see that a drug looks promising but where the confidence interval is very wide, which makes you think that the results are not precise. This might make you interpret the results with caution.

Trying to work through all these different aspects of a trial can be quite challenging if it is not something you do regularly, and so having a framework to help guide you can be very useful.

A range of tools is produced by the Critical Appraisal Skills Programme (CASP) to support you when reading systematic reviews, qualitative analysis or RCTs, to name but a few. You can access these tools online for personal use using the link provided in the references section.

The basis of each of the tools is a series of questions. These act as a framework and are designed to guide you through your thinking about the validity of the piece of work, what the results actually show and whether those results are applicable locally.

Key Points of This Chapter

♦ Evidence-based medicine is about integrating clinical expertise with knowledge of the best available current evidence when making clinical decisions and applying this to your patients.

♦ National guidelines and local formularies can help support evidence-based prescribing and improve patient care as they incorporate the best available evidence about treatments.

♦ Spending on prescribing of both CCGs and individual prescribers is monitored to ensure that prescribing is of high quality and is cost-effective, in that it represents value for money for the whole health economy.

♦ It is difficult to universally ascribe a 'value' to medicines because they are treating human beings. One way of trying to give a value to a medicine, however, is by linking its cost to its health outcomes using quality indices, such as the QALY.

♦ There are a range of different ways that research can be conducted to gather data on pharmaceutical interventions; these are, however, usually conducted using a quantitative methodology such as an RCT.

♦ ARR, RRR and NNT are common statistical ways of presenting results.

♦ To evaluate research, you need to think about the question the research is asking, the design of the study, the results that have been gathered and whether they are applicable to your local population.

Conclusion

Evidence-based medicine is sometimes perceived as a dry subject that has little relevance in day-to-day clinical practice. If you can move past a fear of the statistics, then actually understanding the principles has huge relevance to clinical practice. The reason for this is that how data is collected and interpreted influences what we do for our patients. You have seen in this chapter that the same results can be presented as ARR, RRR and NNT. Even if we are not making the decisions about what is in clinical guidelines or on local formularies, knowing how and why those decisions are made will make you a better-informed prescriber.

References and Further Reading

Aveyard, H. and Sharp, P. (2017) *A Beginner's Guide to Evidence-Based Practice in Health and Social Care*. London: Open University Press.

British Medical Journal (BMJ) BMJ best practice: Fundamentals to learn, practise and discuss EBM. Available at: https://bestpractice.bmj.com/info/toolkit.

Creswell, J. W. and Creswell, J. D. (2018) *Research Design: Qualitative, Quantitative and Mixed Methods Approaches*. London: Sage.

Critical Appraisal Skills Programme (CASP) (2018). CASP checklists. Available at: https://casp-uk.net/casp-tools-checklists.

Ewbank, L., Omojomolo, D., Sullivan, K. et al. (2018) The rising cost of medicines to the NHS: What's the story? London: King's Fund. Available at: https://www.kingsfund.org.uk/sites/default/files/2018-04/Rising-cost-of-medicines.pdf.

Graham, R., Mancher, M., Wolman, D. et al. (2011) *Clinical Practice Guidelines We Can Trust*. Washington DC: National Academics Press.

Greenhalgh, T. (2014) *How to Read a Paper: The Basics of Evidence-based Medicine*. London: Wiley Blackwell.

Hedley, L. and Netto, M. (2013) Cellulitis: What you ought to know. *Pharmaceutical Journal* 291: 193–196.

Mak, V. (2017) Treatment guidelines for COPD – going for GOLD? *Primary Care Respiratory Update* 4(2): 19–24

Moore, A. and McQuay, H. (2006) *Bandolier's Little Book of Making Sense of the Medical Evidence*. Oxford: Oxford University Press.

National Institute for Clinical Excellence (NICE) (2014a) Developing and updating local formularies: Medicines practice guideline [MPG1]. Available at: https://www.nice.org.uk/guidance/mpg1/ https://www.nice.org.uk/process/pmg20/chapter/introduction-and-overview.

National Institute for Clinical Excellence (NICE) (2014b) Developing NICE guidelines: the manual. Process and methods [PMG20]. Available at: https://www.nice.org.uk/process/pmg20/chapter/introduction-and-overview.

National Institute for Clinical Excellence (NICE) (2014c) Patient decision aid: Taking a statin to reduce the risk of coronary heart disease and stroke. Available at: https://www.nice.org.uk/guidance/cg181/resources/patient-decision-aid-pdf-243780159.

National Prescribing Centre (NPC) (2009) *Defining Guiding Principles for Processes Supporting Local Decision Making about Medicines*. London: Department of Health.

Oxford Centre for Evidence-Based Medicine (2009) Oxford Centre for Evidence-Based Medicine – Levels of evidence. Available at: https://www.cebm.net/2009/06/oxford-centre-evidence-based-medicine-levels-evidence-march-2009.

Sackett, D. L., Rosenberg W. M. C., Gray, J. A. et al. (1996) Evidence-based medicine: what it is and what it isn't. *British Medical Journal* 312: 71.

Straus, S. E., Glasziou, P., Richardson, W.S. et al. (2019) *Evidence-Based Medicine: How to Practice and Teach EBM*. Edinburgh: Elsevier.

Chapter 8
Prescribing as Part of a Team

Hannah Ingram

In This Chapter

- Introduction
- Integrated care and healthcare policy
- Integrated care and prescribing practice
- Integrated teamworking
- Clinical governance
- Supplementary prescribing and clinical management plans
- Sharing of information
- Conclusion
- Key points of this chapter
- References and further reading.

Introduction

This chapter explores how the prescribing practice for non-medical prescribers is facilitated in a team-based approach. It also explores clinical governance for independent nurse prescribing, in particular for district nurses. There is a discussion on the use of clinical management plans in supplementary prescribing and also on how information can be shared effectively across teams for safe and effective prescribing practice.

Integrated Care and Healthcare Policy

Healthcare policy in the UK stipulates the need for services to be collaborative and integrated to ensure safe and effective patient care (NHS England 2014, 2019). Integrated care works to address the needs and demands arising in healthcare from an ageing population and increases in people with multi-morbidity. Evidence suggests that integrated approaches to care provide a more positive experience of patients and families in the navigation of health and social care services (Ham and Walsh 2013).

Integrated Care and Prescribing Practice

Integrated care refers not only to services working together to achieve the best outcomes for patients, but also to healthcare professionals working together to ensure effective teamwork. Effective teamworking and the integration of services means that patients receive the 'right care from the right person at the right time' (Charles 2019; NHS Providers 2015). This has meant that in contemporary healthcare practice there has been a development and extension of the roles and responsibilities of healthcare professionals in the development of multi-professional and integrated teams.

In addition, due to fiscal healthcare markets and finite resources in contemporary healthcare, integrated care has meant that professional groups have needed to adopt new roles to maximise their potential in the provision of safe and effective care. District nurses are a great example of healthcare practitioners who have taken on advanced and extended roles, such as independent prescribing, to facilitate timely, safe and effective patient care.

Independent and supplementary prescribing has been a success in contemporary healthcare. It has been able to facilitate timely responses to patient need and a more positive experience of healthcare services for patients and families. This is due to independent prescribers working effectively as part of the wider healthcare team, implementing the principles for effective teamworking within their prescribing practice.

Integrated Team Working

Working as part of a team is essential in prescribing practice, so it is essential for district nurse prescribers to have an awareness that they are not prescribing in isolation, even if some of the specialist work you will be undertaking in practice will mean you are working autonomously. As with your district nursing practice, it is important to remember that in the context of your prescribing practice, you are working as part of a team and that you have a plethora of resources to support you in your prescribing practice.

Principles of Integrated Team Working

The principles of team working include (Nancarrow et al. 2013):

- ◆ Positive leadership
- ◆ Communication
- ◆ Personal rewards
- ◆ Training and development
- ◆ Resources and procedures
- ◆ Skill mix
- ◆ Supportive team climate
- ◆ A shared understanding of roles and objectives
- ◆ Quality outcomes.

Leadership

The principles of teamworking include positive leadership. This may be your responsibility to facilitate within a team, depending on your role. In terms of prescribing practice, you will be a forerunner to district nurse prescribing and will be leading others in the development and evolution of this role, as it develops into specialist practice. In order to facilitate positive leadership in your prescribing practice, it will be useful to reflect on what has gone well, in addition to what you have found a challenge in your prescribing practice, in order to support others coming into the prescribing role.

Communication

Communication is a fundamental aspect of prescribing practice. As an experienced specialist practitioner and district nurse, you will have developed expertise in communication and interaction processes. In terms of your prescribing practice, the focus needs to be on the interaction you have with patients in gaining a concise and holistic health history on which to base a shared prescribing decision. You will need to ensure excellent documentation skills to evidence the rationale for your prescribing decisions and so that any further decisions can be based safely on what you have done.

Personal Rewards

This refers to the value and satisfaction you will feel from prescribing as part of a team, as opposed to any actual physical reward. This will occur as you make prescribing decisions with your patients and are able to realise the difference you have been able to make as part of a team in terms of their care. This may be in diagnosing and/or treating a condition so that the quality of life is improved, or it may be in preventing a hospital admission or in the timely intervention of care.

Training and Development

Ongoing professional development as an independent nurse prescriber is essential. Although once you have your qualification you will need to remain up to date in prescribing practice, you will also have to demonstrate how you maintain currency and competency as part of your NMC revalidation process. Therefore, it is essential that you reflect on your prescribing practice and identify what your ongoing learning needs are. Being part of a wider prescribing team will have its advantages here, as you will be able to learn and share knowledge and experience with other independent prescribers to inform your practice.

Resources and Procedures

These are essential for effective teamworking in prescribing practice. Policy and procedure guidelines will ensure you have robust mechanisms to protect you as a prescriber as well as your patients. Resources needed in prescribing practice will inevitably include time and it is important that, as an independent prescriber, you have the time in practice to undertake thorough assessments and to consider your prescribing decisions in an evidence-based approach with your patients. It will be part of your specialist role to advocate for more time to do this in practice if necessary. Effective communication regarding your learning needs and ongoing development within the wider prescribing team should help facilitate this.

Skill Mix

In the wider integrated team in prescribing practice, each professional will have their own field of expertise. It is essential for integrated care and safe and effective prescribing that this is shared. Other professionals will want to access your expertise from your district nursing practice, and you may need their help at other times. Open and honest communication about your skills, knowledge and experience and your scope of prescribing practice will ensure that the patient is treated by the right person and that no undue pressure is placed upon you to prescribe in an area where you do not have the competence to do so.

Supportive Team Climate

By undertaking the principles of integrated teamworking, a collaborative approach to prescribing practice will be evident. Support is a multi-way concept in prescribing practice, and as an independent prescriber, you will find that you will be providing support to other independent and supplementary prescribers as well as seeking it for yourself. It is essential to remember when you start prescribing that it is a new and complex role.

Asking for help when it is needed is crucial – other prescribers have been where you are and will support any learning and development needs you have. All independent prescribers, from whatever discipline, remember their first encounter with a patient that resulted in prescribing activity, and the nerves, fear and satisfaction that came with this. Integrated care incorporates valuing each other as practitioners; this is particularly true in prescribing practice, and independent and supplementary prescribers will work hard to support each other.

A Shared Understanding of Roles and Objectives

This is essential in prescribing practice. It is imperative that other people understand your role, your prescribing role and your scope of prescribing practice. Likewise, it is essential that you have a clear understanding of the roles of the other professionals you are working with. This allows for clear boundaries and reduces the unrealistic expectations on your practice that can cause conflict.

As a district nurse, you will be working as part of a larger team and this is likely to include a leadership role where you support and manage junior team members. Once you are an independent prescriber, it is likely that your team of junior staff will come to you requesting prescriptions for patients on your caseload, rather than seek these out from a GP, as accessing you will be quicker and easier for them.

It is important to remember that as a district nurse independent prescriber, it is not your role to make up for the shortfall that may exist in other services, such as general practice. **You should only prescribe when you can demonstrate safe and effective decision making**. This means that best practice, when prescribing, is to undertake a full and comprehensive assessment yourself on which to base your decision making, rather than relying on the assessment of junior staff. You will need to justify your decision making to yourself, your employer, the patient and the NMC should this be called into question. Therefore, this is a serious issue to consider. This can be challenging when there are limited resources in community nursing and time is at a premium, but always remember that not only will your prescribing qualification be called into question should there be a negative patient outcome, but so will your overall registration. The two cannot be separated. Therefore, always be sure of your decision making, that it is based on a full and comprehensive health assessment, that you can justify your actions and that you can demonstrate safe and effective person-centred prescribing.

Case Study 8.1

District nurse new independent prescriber Sarah was asked by her team to prescribe antibiotics for a patient on the caseload by a staff nurse at handover. Due to pressure in practice, a good relationship with the staff nurse and a reasonable knowledge of the patient, Sarah considered doing this. Sarah questioned the experienced staff nurse, who reported the clinical symptoms of cellulitis. Sarah considered prescribing flucloxacillin, the BNF (2019) and local first-line treatment for cellulitis, and went on to think about drug interactions and allergies for the patient. Establishing that she did not have adequate information, she decided not to prescribe at this time, but went to review the patient herself to ascertain this information before making a final prescribing decision or liaising with the patient's GP.

On assessing the patient, Sarah's assessment established that the patient was experiencing varicose eczema, was on warfarin and had an allergy to penicillin.

Had Sarah prescribed on the nurse's assessment, this would have put the patient at risk and been an inappropriate use of antibiotic therapy.

Quality Outcomes

Undertaking safe and effective evidence-based prescribing practice will support quality outcomes in patient care, and in turn will boost your confidence and competence as a prescriber and will develop effective integrated team working.

Turn to **Chapter 9** for more on the legal and ethical aspects of prescribing, **Chapter 2** for more detail about consultation and patient-centred approaches to care, **Chapter 3** for theories on decision making and **Chapter 12** for suggestions about undertaking consistent and useful reflective activity.

Clinical Governance

Patient safety is paramount in prescribing practice, and as such district nurses must prescribe within the law and strive to continually improve their practice to benefit patient care (RCN 2019).

Governance structures will be in place if you are employed within NHS and social care organisations, and these must be adhered to as an independent prescriber. Governance structures for prescribing practice should include:

♦ Clear lines of responsibility and accountability and that this is evidenced in your job description
♦ Development of quality improvement structures such as supporting evidence-based practice, audit (ePACT data)
♦ Access continuing professional development (CPD) as required
♦ Risk management strategies, policies and procedures are in place
♦ Regularly engage in prescribing supervision and prescribing governance meetings
♦ Poor performance procedures are in place and that you are able to report poor performance or concerns related to prescribing practice
♦ Competency frameworks for prescribing are utilised for regular self-assessment (RPS 2016)
♦ Prescribe from local agreed formularies
♦ Demonstrate the responsibilities and processes of ensuring safe care of prescription pads
♦ Record prescribing decisions contemporaneously and in line with your organisational policy
♦ Ensure collaborative working with the wider integrated healthcare team
♦ Report any restrictions to practice or change in health and good character that may impact on your ability to prescribe safely and effectively.

Audit

Audit is an essential part of your prescribing practice. If you are practising as both an independent and supplementary prescriber, each role should be audited separately. Supplementary prescribers should ensure that they meet at least annually with the medical prescriber to review prescribing practice. You should also undertake an audit as a supplementary prescriber to see how many clinical management plans have been followed correctly.

Audit processes should include how many patients you have prescribed for required medical follow-up and how many have been successfully treated. It is also good practice to audit the number of patients you decided not to prescribe for or to de-prescribe for, and the outcomes of these prescribing encounters. You can also audit how many times a pharmacist has had to contact you regarding the clarity of a prescription you have issued, which will inform your reflective and prescribing practice.

Feedback from patients on your prescribing practice is useful for your reflection and CPD. It is helpful to have feedback from patients for appraisal purposes and to develop your prescribing practice when things have not gone so well, but it is also confidence-building when positive feedback is received.

Supplementary Prescribing and Clinical Management Plans

Nurses who hold the independent prescribing qualification and annotation with the NMC will also be annotated as supplementary prescribers. If you are prescribing as a supplementary prescriber, you will be prescribing in a team context with a medical prescriber (doctor or dentist).

If you are prescribing as a supplementary prescriber, you must do so within the limits of a clinical management plan (CMP) for an individual patient. A CMP allows you to prescribe certain medicines for certain medical conditions for individual patients in collaboration and partnership with a medical prescriber. CMPs must be written with you, as the supplementary prescriber, and the medical doctor you are collaborating with, and you must have the patient's consent. As a supplementary prescriber, you must never prescribe outside of a CMP. If you are a nurse independent prescriber and supplementary prescriber, you must adhere to the CMP when prescribing as a supplementary prescriber. This does not stop you from prescribing for this patient for an unrelated condition as an independent prescriber within your scope of practice. If you are prescribing for a certain condition, then this prescribing activity will need to remain within the CMP as a supplementary prescriber, as **Case Study 8.2** highlights.

The CMP must be recorded before you begin prescribing. This can be a signed paper version or an electronic record. Should the CMP need to be modified, this must be done in partnership with you as the supplementary prescriber

> ## Case Study 8.2
>
> You are prescribing for Mrs Jones as a nurse supplementary prescriber under a CMP for her COPD (as this is a new area to your scope of prescribing practice).
>
> However, during a consultation, you diagnose a urinary tract infection (UTI).
>
> You can treat the UTI as an independent prescriber, if prescribing for low-grade infections and antibiotic prescribing is within the scope of your prescribing practice.

and with the medical prescriber; this is also the case should the CMP need to be discontinued in light of any change to the patient status. As the district nurse supplementary prescriber, you have a responsibility to refer back to the medical prescriber with any change in the patient's condition.

Sharing of Information

Prescribing is not an activity that ever happens in isolation. You will be making shared decisions where possible with patients. You must also share the information regarding your prescribing decisions and activity with other practitioners involved in the care who will benefit from the information. You will need to think carefully of the best way to share this information and you will need to consider the General Data Protection Regulation (GDPR) and the Data Protection Act (HM Government 2018) in the sharing of information.

Ideally, you will have access to contemporary records and to other practitioners' prescribing records, but in practice this is not always the case. IT systems across the NHS rarely 'speak to each other', so it is important that you communicate your prescribing decisions to the appropriate people to ensure the patient's safety and explore all avenues to ensure you have the most up-to-date information on which to base your prescribing decisions.

You must have the patient's consent to share information with other healthcare professionals, and you must explain to them that your prescribing activity cannot be taken in isolation of the wider healthcare team (RPS 2016). If the patient refuses to give consent, you should fully explain the risks involved of not communicating your prescribing actions. If the patient continues to refuse, you must consider the best course of action to ensure the patient's safety. This may be to not prescribe. You must document your decision in the patient's notes (RPS 2016).

Conclusion

This chapter has highlighted that prescribing practice for district nurses is an integrated approach to care and that prescribing does not happen in isolation. As an independent nurse prescriber, you are prescribing as part of a wider healthcare team and should work to ensure that a collaborative approach to care is facilitated with good team working. As a prescriber, you will need to ensure that clinical governance is maintained to safeguard quality in your prescribing practice.

As a novice independent nurse prescriber, you may wish to undertake supplementary prescribing in collaboration with a medical prescriber, and to do this you must remain within the limits of a clinical management plan and ensure team working with the medical prescriber and the patient.

The sharing of information is essential in prescribing practice in order to ensure patient safety. This needs to occur in a contemporaneous way and with the patient's consent. Data protection should be considered when sharing information.

Key Points of This Chapter

♦ This role you are about to undertake is very important and can be risky. It is vital to access assistance and help as you require it from the multi-professional team and use the support that is available.
♦ Use the CMPs as you have been taught.
♦ Reflect on and review your prescribing practice via audit and any other mechanism which will assist you to continue growing in confidence and competence.

References and Further Reading

British National Formulary (BNF) (2019) *The British National Formulary 75: March – September 2019.* London: The BMJ Group.

Charles, A. (2019). *Community Services Explained.* London: The King's Fund.

Ham, C. and Walsh, N. (2013) *Making Integrated Care Happen at Scale and Pace.* London: The King's Fund.

HM Government (2018) *Data Protection Act.* London: The Stationery Office.

Nancarrow, S. A., Booth, A., Ariss, S. et al. (2013) Ten principles of good interdisciplinary team work. *Human Resources for Health* 11(19). Available at: https://www.ncbi.nlm. nih.gov/pmc/articles/PMC3662612/pdf/1478-4491-11-19.pdf (last accessed 20 June).

NHS England (2014) *The Five Year Forward View.* London: NHS England.

NHS England (2019) *The NHS Long Term Plan.* London: NHS England.

NHS Providers (2015) *Right Place, Right Time, Better Transfers of Care: A Call to Action.* London: Association of NHS Providers Foundation Trusts and Trusts.

Royal College of Nursing (RCN) (2019) Non-medical prescribing. Available at: https://www.rcn.org.uk/get-help/rcn-advice/non-medical-prescribers (last accessed 20 June).

Royal Pharmaceutical Society (RPS) (2016) *A Competency Framework for All Prescribers.* London: Royal Pharmaceutical Society.

Chapter 9
Law and Ethics

Hannah Ingram

In This Chapter

- ◆ Introduction
- ◆ Prescribing
- ◆ Scope of prescribing practice
- ◆ Indemnity insurance
- ◆ Licensing
- ◆ Legal considerations
- ◆ Ethical considerations
- ◆ Good practice considerations
- ◆ Controlled drugs
- ◆ Evidence-based prescribing
- ◆ Conclusion
- ◆ Key points of this chapter
- ◆ References and further reading.

Introduction

This chapter will outline the legislation and legal aspects that support you as district nurse independent prescribers in practice. Key legal and ethical concepts related to prescribing practice will be explored, as well as utilising evidence-based practice for safe and effective prescribing practice.

Prescribing

Prescribing is defined as the advice and authorisation to use a medicine from the British National Formulary (BNF), and often includes the writing and issuing of a prescription (HCPC 2018).

Due to the nature of district nursing, it is likely that you may be handwriting your prescriptions in the patient's home for immediate access to medicines, when there is an appropriate person available to arrange collection from a dispensing pharmacy. When a prescription is written by hand, you must make sure that this written legibly, unambiguously, in ink, dated and with the full name, address and date of birth of the patient. This should of course be signed by you, the prescribing practitioner (once you are legally annotated with the NMC to prescribe). The age of the patient must be legally stated on a prescription if it is for a child under 12 years old (BNF 2019). This is to ensure prescriptions are complete and meet the legal requirements (RPS 2016).

There are differing legal systems that govern prescribing throughout each country in the UK and as independent prescribers, district nurses should be familiar with local legal systems. The primary legislation that allows nurses to prescribe is the Medicinal Products: Prescription by Nurses and Others Act 1992. A nurse is defined as a registered nurse, health visitor or midwife in Chapter 28, Article 1.

Since the inception of nurse prescribing in 1992, there have been many adjustments to the legislation and to the titles of nurse prescribing roles and annotations within the NMC to reflect changes in contemporary nursing practice.

Nurse prescribing was initiated in the community for district nurses, as discussed in the background chapter of this book. Currently, there are three annotations of nurse prescribing that are recordable with the NMC which have formed part of the legislation since 2006 (RCN 2019).

The V100 refers to the nurse prescribing qualification that is acquired by district nurses or public health nurses (formally known as health visitors (RCN 2019)), as part of a Specialist Practitioner qualification. This allows these nurses to prescribe for the Nurse Prescribers' Formulary (NPF) within their scope of practice, on successful completion of the relevant education programme. These nurses must not only complete the V100 module as part of the Specialist Practitioner course but must also successfully complete the Specialist Practitioner course itself before the prescribing qualification is recordable with the NMC and they can then go on to prescribe (NMC 2018).

The V150 refers to a nurse prescribing qualification that community nurses can take as a stand-alone education programme (e.g. not part of a wider course) that allows them, on successful completion, to prescribe within their scope of practice from the NPF.

The NPF is a formulary of medicines and preparations for community practitioner nurse prescribers (district nurses and public health nurses) which provides details of preparations that can be prescribed for patients receiving NHS treatment on a community prescription form (NPAG 2017), such as an FP10 in England; other UK nations have their own codes for community prescriptions and these can be sourced in the NPF or the British National Formulary (BNF).

Community practitioner nurse prescribers, those with a V100 and V150 annotated NMC qualification, must prescribe only from the list of preparations in the NPF for the conditions listed in the NPF, and these should be prescribed generically unless it is stipulated in the formulary that a brand name can be used. The

NPF is formulated by the Nurse Prescribers' Advisory Group and is regularly reviewed based on nurse prescriber feedback, the medicines and preparations available and the evidence base available.

The V300 is the NMC annotation that refers to independent and supplementary nurse prescribers.

In English law there are two types of prescribers who can prescribe medicines from the BNF. These are independent prescribers and supplementary prescribers; see **Boxes 9.1** and **9.2** for definitions.

In England, further changes to medicines legislation in 2006 allowed nurses to become independent and supplementary prescribers following a post-registration education programme that is approved by the NMC. Until 2019 this was in conjunction with the NMC's (2006) standards of proficiency for nurse and midwife prescribers and has now been superseded by the *Competency Framework for all Prescribers* (RPS 2016), and the new standard for nurse prescribing which is Part 3 of the NMC's *Realising Professionalism: Standards for Education and Training, Standards for Prescribing Programmes* (NMC 2019).

Box 9.1 – Definition of independent prescribers

Independent prescribers are those who are accountable and responsible for the assessment and treatment of new or previously diagnosed conditions and the decisions made as part of a clinical treatment plan, which may include prescribing (BNF 2017). Independent prescribers can prescribe, stop or adjust any medicine from the BNF for patients in their care within their scope of practice.

Box 9.2 – Definition of supplementary prescribers

Supplementary prescribers work in partnership with a medical prescriber (such as a doctor or a dentist) and can implement the commencement, titration or de-prescribing of certain medicines for pre-determined patients within a clinical management plan, with the patients' consent (BNF 2017). This means that supplementary prescribers can prescribe a range of identified medicines for certain patients within their scope of practice, with the support of a medical prescriber who writes a clinical management plan for the supplementary prescriber to follow.

The prescribing award obtained must be registered with the NMC within five years of successful completion. If it is not, then it will have to be taken again in its entirety to successfully complete and qualify as a prescriber. Prescribing can only take place once the qualification has been annotated to the NMC register, and prescribing can only be undertaken from the formulary that the qualification covers and within the scope of practice and competence of the nurse prescriber (NMC 2018).

The NMC's standards for proficiency for nurse and midwife prescribers (NMC 2006) remain available as a reference source; however, nurse prescribers must NOT use these to inform their ongoing practice, but rather should refer to the RPS (2016) *Competency Framework* to do so, in line with the standard for nurse prescribing which is Part 3 of the NMC's *Realising Professionalism: Standards for Education and Training, Standards for Prescribing Programmes* (NMC 2018), as well as other relevant resources (NMC 2019).

Only once the prescribing education programme is successfully completed can the nurse annotate their prescribing qualification against their NMC registration in order to practise as a prescriber (NMC 2018). Prescribing practice can only commence when the prescribing qualification is visible on the NMC register with no restrictions, and there is support and indemnity insurance in place with the employer to prescribe. Independent prescribing status allows nurses to prescribe any medicine from the BNF as long as this is within the competence and scope of practice of the prescriber.

Education programmes approved by the NMC include training and preparation in competencies to undertake independent and supplementary prescribing. Therefore, if you are annotated as an independent nurse prescriber on the NMC register, you will also be annotated as a supplementary prescriber (RCN 2019). This may be of use when you are developing your scope of prescribing practice into new disease areas or in prescribing a new range of drugs. Using a clinical management plan as a supplementary prescriber could also be of use to you should you move into a new role or speciality and take your prescribing qualification with you. This will help you develop a new scope of prescribing practice in a new field of practice in a supportive context.

Scope of Prescribing Practice

Independent and supplementary prescribing for nurses was introduced to support and enhance the delivery of care to patients in a range of healthcare settings, and will be undertaken by nurses in specialist or advanced roles. If a district nurse is working in their specialist role, it does not mean they are 'entitled to be' or 'should be' independent prescribers.

The role being undertaken by the specialist practitioner district requires consideration to ascertain if independent prescribing is an essential part of the role and if it therefore should be part of the job description. Where prescribing is identified as an essential aspect of the clinical role, the district nurses will be required to undertake an accredited postgraduate independent prescribing course at a higher education institution in order to achieve the qualification (NMC 2018; RCN 2019).

As a specialist practitioner district nurse, you may have undertaken the V100 prescribing qualification and now wish to expand your scope of prescribing practice and undertake the V300 independent prescribing qualification. This will need to be deemed appropriate by your employer and there should be an identified need for you to prescribe in practice. District nurses can hold both prescribing qualifications. Although the principles of prescribing practice may be the same, the scope of prescribing practice will be different and therefore new knowledge and the application of new knowledge is required. In addition, the new NMC prescribing standards stipulate that prescribing programmes must incorporate the *Competency Framework for all Prescribers* (RPS 2016) and you may not have encountered this as part of your V100 qualification; therefore, the V300 educational programme should be completed in its entirety. Programme providers may consider recognition of prior learning that is capable of being mapped against the RPS (2016) *Competency Framework for all Prescribers* (NMC 2018).

Contemporary district nursing practice suggests that independent prescribing is becoming increasingly essential for district nursing practice. The new *District Nurse Apprenticeship Standard* (Institute for Apprenticeship and Technical Education 2019) states that the Specialist Practice qualifications of district nursing should now have independent prescribing integral to the education programme.

Your scope of prescribing practice will relate to the areas in which you are safe and competent to prescribe. Your personal scope of prescribing practice should be identified with your employer and non-medical or independent prescribing lead. As a district nurse independent prescriber, you should identify which groups of patients you will be prescribing for, such as adults or older people.

This relates to your scope of prescribing practice, and you should only prescribe for those groups where you have expertise and competence and where it is agreed with your employer you are able to prescribe. With the development of new ways of working and the integration of healthcare services, there can be an expectation that skills are transferrable to other areas of practice (NHS England 2014, 2019). For example, if a district nurse is asked to prescribe for a child, this should be referred on to another prescriber as this would be working outside of their area of expertise and competence (NICE 2019b; RCN 2019).

As a district nurse independent prescriber, you will also need to identify which conditions you will be treating within your scope of prescribing practice. This can be quite generic for district nursing practice as it is a specialist generalist role. However, depending on service delivery models, this may become quite specific if you are working in a particular speciality such as palliative care.

Your scope of practice may include diabetes, COPD, low-grade infection management and skin conditions. You would then need to identify the group of medicines you intend to use within your scope of prescribing practice: for example, antidiabetic medication, inhalers and steroids, antibiotics, emollients, steroid creams and ointments.

An example of a scope of prescribing practice document is provided in **Figure 9.1**; however, each organisation will have its own. It is important to include one of these in your supervision or appraisal processes as a new district nurse prescriber. You can review your scope of prescribing practice as your confidence and competence in prescribing develops. You are not limited to the disease areas of medicines you identify at the start of your prescribing practice, and this will develop as your scope of prescribing practice does. You should only ever prescribe medicines that you have an in-depth understanding of and are competent to prescribe, and that are within your scope of prescribing

Scope of prescribing practice		
Prescriber's name		
Job title		
Disease area(s) you will be prescribing for (Please list)		
Age group(s) you will be prescribing for (Tick as appropriate)	Neonates	
	Children and young people	
	Adults	
	Elderly	
Groups of medicines you will be prescribing (Please list)		

Prescriber's signature...
Date ....

Manager/Non-Medical Prescribing (NMP) lead signature.......................
Date ....

Figure 9.1 – Example of a scope of prescribing practice document

practice. You should not feel obliged to prescribe anything you do not have a comprehensive knowledge of, even if this has been prescribed for your patient previously, especially if it is outside of your scope of prescribing practice, as you will be accountable for this action.

> **Key point!**
>
> You must only prescribe in the areas in which you are knowledgeable and skilled to do so safely.
>
> You must also only prescribe in the areas in which your employer has agreed that you can do so, where this is safe to do so and you have the required employee and prescribing insurances in place.

As a district nurse and independent prescriber, your role is to continue to facilitate multi-professional working in the care of patients. This should be done within your professional role and core competency, and prescribing for patients should not be done to make up for a 'shortfall' in other prescribers in practice settings, such as an inability to obtain a GP visit or a lack of specialist resources. You should be able to recognise and manage factors that may unduly influence your prescribing practice (RPS 2016).

Your prescribing practice and trends can also be reviewed using a scope of prescribing practice document, similar to the example shown in **Figure 9.1**. Of course, you can and should review and reflect on your own practice, but it will be reviewed during your appraisal process and prescribing practice review, when exploring your ePACT prescribing data.

>
> Turn to **Chapter 11** for more detail regarding medicines optimisation.

As an independent nurse prescriber, your scope of prescribing practice must fall within the scope of district nursing practice and be based on your practice setting. You must know and work within the legal and regulatory frameworks for your prescribing practice, and make decisions based on patient need and not your personal considerations (RPS 2016).

Indemnity Insurance

Nurses working in clinical practice have to have indemnity insurance to protect the public and themselves. As an independent prescriber, this insurance will need to cover your prescribing practice. Indemnity insurance as a prescriber may be provided within your employment contract or you may have to source this separately. For your safety and that of your patients, it is essential that you are clear on this for your role before you commence prescribing.

If you are employed, you should not have to organise separate indemnity insurance as your employer should have vicarious liability insurance. This means that they as your employer are responsible for your actions and omissions at work, and as such should provide indemnity cover for you. This applies if you work for the NHS or a private employer and it is inappropriate for your employer to shift this responsibility onto you or your union (RCN 2019a). This includes if you are prescribing or working independently in a specialist area (such as district nursing); you should not have to top up this insurance to cover your prescribing practice. However, to ensure that these insurances are valid, you need to ensure that prescribing is part of your job description and person specification, that you are fully supported by your employer to prescribe, that you only prescribe within your scope of practice and competence, and that there are no restrictions on your practice.

If you are self-employed, you need to arrange your own indemnity insurance. In the UK, district nurses are employed and therefore private indemnity insurance is not needed. However, if you are undertaking other work on a self-employed basis, such as aesthetics, then you will need indemnity insurance to cover this practice and ensure that it covers prescribing practice specifically. It is important to note that RCN members have indemnity insurance in their membership, but that since 2014 this has not included aesthetics practice (RCN 2019a).

To undertake prescribing practice, and for the insurance to be valid, you must hold a valid prescribing qualification and be annotated as a prescriber on the NMC register. Therefore, you are not permitted to prescribe until your prescribing qualification has been annotated and is visible on the NMC register.

The Human Medicines Regulations (2012) provides an update to the Medicines Act (1968). These law statutes ensure that the evaluation and manufacture of medicines, and the sale and supply of medicines are regulated to keep people as safe as possible. The Human Medicines Regulations (HMR) also classify medicines for supply. These are detailed in Table 9.1.

Licensing

The Medicines and Healthcare Products Regulatory Authority (MHRA) is an executive agency that regulates the medicines, medical devices and blood components for transfusion in the UK. It provides a valid marketing authorisation for the use of medicines in the UK. This valid marketing authorisation was formally known as a Product Licence. This gives a medicine a licence for use in its indicated treatments.

Table 9.1 – The Human Medicines Regulations classification of medicines for supply

General Sales List (GSL) Medicines A GSL medicine is deemed by the licensing authority to be on general sale. These medicines do not require a prescription or supervision from a pharmacist to be sold and are readily available in retail outlets. Examples are paracetamol and ibuprofen.
Pharmacy (P) Medicines This category of medicines can be sold without a prescription, but only under the supervision of a pharmacist. Examples are hydrocortisone 1% and co-codomol.
Prescription Only Medicines (POMs) These medicines are only available on prescription from a recognised and professionally annotated prescriber. Examples are amoxicillin and fluoxetine.
Patient Group Directions (PGDs) A PGD is not a classification of a medicine, but an exemption of how medicines can be supplied. This is a written direction that relates to the 'sale, supply and administration of a description or class of medicinal product' (HM Government 2012). A PGD enables named, authorised and registered health professionals to administer medicines to pre-defined groups of patients without a prescription so that patents have safe and speedy access to the medicines they need. A PGD should be drawn up by a multi-professional group, including a medical prescriber (doctor or dentist) and a pharmacist, with representation from the professional group who will be administering medicines under the PGD, such as a nurse or paramedic (England 2016).
Patient Specific Directions (PSDs) A PSD is a written instruction by a registered and annotated prescribing professional for medicines to be supplied and/or administered to a named patient. It can be completed by an independent district nurse prescriber and may include drug authorisation charts (England 2016).

There are some exemptions from licensing within the MHRA; these include herbal remedies, the import and supply of unlicensed relevant medicinal products for individual patients and the manufacture and supply of unlicensed medicine products for individual patients, known as 'specials' (MHRA 2019; NMC 2006). Further information can be found on the MHRA website: https://www.gov.uk/government/organisations/medicines-and-healthcare-products-regulatory-agency.

As independent prescribers, district nurses will be able to prescribe any licensed medicine for any medical condition within their competence and scope of practice.

From 2008, independent nurse prescribers have been able to issue private prescriptions for any licensed medicines that they are competent to prescribe, excepting ALL controlled drugs; however, it is recommended that professional indemnity insurance is held if prescribing outside of the NHS (RCN 2019a).

Unlicensed Use

Unlicensed drugs refer to medicines that do not hold an MHRA valid marketing authorisation but are listed in the BNF. In general, the BNF will only list medicines that are supported by a valid marketing authorisation. Where there is an unlicensed medicine in the BNF, this is indicated in square brackets after the entry (BNF 2018). Independent district nurse prescribers are permitted to independently prescribe unlicensed medicines, and medicines for use outside of their licence (off-label). However, as an independent prescriber, this must be within your clinical competence, your professional code and the terms of your employment (NICE 2014).

Prescribing an unlicensed medicine and prescribing off-label increases risk and increases responsibility as a prescriber. The risks may include (NICE 2014):

- Adverse reactions
- Poor product quality
- Lack of product information and poor labelling
- Patient information leaflets do not concur with the use you have prescribed it for.

However, as an independent district nurse prescriber, you may wish to prescribe as a supplementary prescriber and use an unlicensed medicine in a clinical management plan in collaboration with a GP. See below for NICE (2014) guidance on this process.

Off-label

The term 'off-label' refers to the use of a medicine that has a valid marketing authorisation, but is administered via a route (e.g. sublingual, orally, rectally) or method that is outside of the licensed indication of the product. Therefore, off-label prescribing is where a licensed medicine is prescribed outside of its licence. There are a number of circumstances where as independent prescribers nurses can prescribe off-label, but this is most likely to be when prescribing for children and therefore is not appropriate for district nurses as this is outside of their scope of practice.

As a district nurse independent prescriber, you may legally prescribe medicines off-label, but you must accept clinical, professional and legal responsibility for doing so. You must make sure that the following conditions of prescribing off-label are met.

NICE (2014) guidance for prescribers in prescribing off-label or unlicensed medicines is as follows:

♦ Be satisfied that an alternative, licensed medicine would not meet the patient's needs before prescribing an unlicensed medicine
♦ Be satisfied that such use would better serve the patient's needs than an appropriately licensed alternative before prescribing a medicine off-label
♦ Before prescribing an unlicensed medicine or using a medicine off-label you should:
  ◗ e satisfied that there is a sufficient evidence base and/or experience of using the medicine to show its safety and efficacy
  ◗ Take responsibility for prescribing the medicine and for overseeing the patient's care, including monitoring and follow-up
  ◗ Record the medicine prescribed and, where common practice is not being followed, the reasons for prescribing this medicine; you may wish to record that you have discussed the issue with the patient.

Best practice for communication includes:

♦ You give patients, or those authorising treatment on their behalf, sufficient information about the proposed treatment, including known serious or common adverse reactions, to enable them to make an informed decision.
♦ Where current practice supports the use of a medicine outside the terms of its licence, it may not be necessary to draw attention to the licence when seeking consent. However, it is good practice to give as much information as patients or carers require or which they may see as relevant.
♦ You explain the reasons for prescribing a medicine off-label or prescribing an unlicensed medicine where there is little evidence to support its use, or where the use of a medicine is innovative.

An example of prescribing off-label: metformin is licensed for use in diabetes. It is also accepted clinical practice to use metformin in the treatment for polycystic ovary syndrome; however, the marketing authorisation does not include polycystic ovary syndrome in its indications of use. Therefore, prescribing metformin for polycystic ovary syndrome would be off-label.

It is often necessary to prescribe off-label in paediatric practice as medicines are often not licensed for use in children. This is due to the lack of clinical trials undertaken in children due to ethical reasons. You must explain any off-label prescribing to parents or guardians and apply the same principles for prescribing in adults. You must also refer to the BNF for children and other appropriate guidelines before making any decisions in prescribing for children.

Legal Considerations

There are legal and ethical considerations to independent prescribing for district nurses. As an experienced practitioner taking on independent prescribing within your role, you will be very familiar with the legal and ethical considerations for your practice. It is worth further consideration to reflect on how prescribing practice may influence and impact on these considerations.

Accountability

As a professional and as an independent prescriber, you are accountable for your own prescribing decisions; this includes all actions and omissions. This accountability cannot be delegated and you will be fully responsible for all of the prescribing process. You must only prescribe within your own scope of practice, competence and experience, and in line with the NMC standards and code for professional conduct and the RPS (2016) competency framework. As an independent nurse prescriber, you must demonstrate competence and evidence to support your ongoing prescribing practice in line with the NMC code and RPS (2016) competency framework for your professional registration revalidation.

As an independent nurse prescriber, you must only prescribe for patients who you have assessed and for whom you have made the prescribing decision. You should inform patients that you are an independent non-medical district nurse prescriber, that you can only prescribe within your scope of prescribing practice and that there may be some circumstances when you need to refer on to another professional. In primary care, you should only prescribe using an FP10 prescription pad which has your own individual NMC number on it. Accountability for the prescription is with the prescriber who has prescribed the medicines.

Most NHS organisations now use local formularies in practice. This is to ensure evidence-based and cost-efficient prescribing practice. Some NHS organisations will only allow you to prescribe within this formulary, despite your independent prescribing status; some will allow you to prescribe outside of the formulary if you are able to demonstrate a clear rationale for doing so. Any restrictions placed on you through a formulary would only apply while you are working with that employer.

If you move practice area or move to work with a new employer, you may need to undertake further training and education if you wish to prescribe in a new speciality. Your new employer may wish to assess your competency as a prescriber before they support your prescribing in practice. If you undertake prescribing practice outside of employment, for example as an independent practitioner in the aesthetics industry, you will need to ensure you have completed the full training required and hold your own indemnity insurance. You will need to ensure you have the skills, knowledge and competence to prescribe in this area before doing so. If your practice or prescribing practice is called into question outside of your regular independent district nurse prescribing role, this will have implications for all your practice roles.

If there are any restrictions placed on your practice by the NMC, it is your responsibility to inform your employer and/or insurance providers of any implications this may have on your ability to prescribe in practice.

Consent

You must explain your role as an independent nurse prescriber to the patient. You will need to explain that you are able to prescribe within your own scope of prescribing practice and that there may be circumstances where you will need to refer them on to another healthcare professional. You should provide the patient with all the information regarding your prescribing decision so that they are able to provide informed consent to any treatment. You should also adhere to any employer or local guidelines on gaining consent in practice for treatment.

Using a patient-centred approach to prescribing, you should be aware of any social, religious or cultural factors that may impact on a patient's choice of treatment and that may affect your prescribing decisions. For example, vegetarians will not want gelatine-based capsules.

As discussed earlier, when considering off-label prescribing, you must clearly explain to the patient if you are prescribing outside of the marketing authorisation. If you are prescribing a medication in a way that is not specified on the Summary of Product Characteristics or manufacturer's data sheets, then this is off-licence/off-label prescribing and the patient needs to be fully informed in order to give their consent to treatment. The patient has a right to refuse any treatment you may wish to prescribe for them; however, if they do, you need to explain the risks and potential outcomes of this decision so that they are fully informed.

(Breach of) Duty of Care

As a nurse and as a prescriber, you have a duty of care to your patients. A duty of care is to provide the best care based on the best evidence available in a timely and professional way, causing no harm. Once a duty of care has been established, it needs to be demonstrated that the practitioner caused a breach of duty of care. The actions and/or omissions of the practitioner will need to be explored to ascertain if they reached the accepted level of competence. In order for this to occur, the practitioner's actions are judged by the standards of their peers in the same role. This is the legal standing in the UK decided following the landmark case *Bolam v Friern Hospital Management Committee* (1957).

Negligence

Negligence is the neglect of care of a patient. Negligence in prescribing practice is the failing to provide a duty of care, failing to exercise reasonable care, or the breach of duty resulting in poor or adverse outcomes for the patient.

Failing to provide adequate information on a medicine you prescribe or failing to undertake a thorough and holistic patient assessment as part of your consultation could result in negligence of your patient. It is negligent in law to fail to communicate appropriately (Dimond 2015). You will need to ensure that not only do you communicate all the required information to the patient, but that your record-keeping reflects this discussion. Prescribing is a complex and potentially risky activity. You need to ensure that you are prescribing within your scope of prescribing practice, that you are clinically competent, skilled and knowledgeable to do so, and that your prescribing decision is based on the best available evidence and is made in partnership with your patient.

Ethical Considerations

In considering an ethical approach to prescribing practice, it is essential to consider the ethical principles of Beauchamp and Childress (2013). There are other models for ethical practice that can be accessed by nurse prescribers for consideration.

Autonomy

Autonomy is to respect the patient's right to choose. There is a focus in contemporary healthcare practice on facilitating a patient-centred, shared decision-making approach to ensure the patient's voice is heard and they are able to make informed decisions about their care. It is essential, therefore, that this is incorporated into prescribing consultations and decision making. As a district nurse prescriber, you will need to respect the decisions of your patients to refuse or decline treatment that you would like to initiate, or to choose a different course of action. It is essential that you ensure the patient has the information with which to make an informed decision and is aware of the potential outcomes should they not take your advice. You will also need to ensure that this information is clearly documented in the patient notes. The use of Patient Information Sheets, available with medicines, may help patients reach an informed decision on the proposed course of action. It is important to remember that declining your intervention does not necessary indicate a lack of capacity to choose (Department of Constitutional Affairs 2005), but may reflect choice based on health beliefs and experience, and this should be explored with the patient.

Non-maleficence

This is the principle that outlines the concept to 'do no harm'. You will consider any adverse effects that the medicine you wish to prescribe may have and will fully inform the patient of these. In a patient-centred and shared decision-making approach, you will need to weigh up the risk-benefit ratio of commencing a medication with potential adverse effects, using your expertise and patient choice. You will also have the ethical duty to consider any potential interactions that adding a new medication to the patient's medication regime may have.

Beneficence

This is the ethical principle of 'doing good' and is central of the professional district nursing role and healthcare practice. In undertaking this process, you will be ensuring that you are seeking out the best available prescribing option for your patient as an individual. This will be based on a person-centred holistic assessment and the best available evidence. It is imperative to ensure a patient-centred approach to this ethical principle so that you are not paternalistic in your prescribing practice, but are able to work in partnership with your patients, ensuring autonomy and shared decision making.

Justice

This is the ethical principle of 'fairness', although the breadth of justice in healthcare is much wider than this. In fiscal healthcare markets it is essential as a prescriber that district nurses consider the cost implications of individual prescribing decisions and the wider cost of prescribing. This can include considering prescribing within formularies, contributing to the development of formularies and considering if medicine use is effective for the patients you care for. It is important to remember that justice in contemporary healthcare can be distributive justice. This includes ensuring that your prescribing practice is cost-effective so that resources are sustainable. The overriding principle is that resources should be available to all on point of need. For example, you may advise a patient to purchase paracetamol over the counter rather than prescribe it, as this is a more cost-effective and sustainable option.

Good Practice Considerations

It is essential to consider 'good practice' elements of prescribing practice when considering the legal and ethical implications of practice.

You must never prescribe for yourself. This would not be a legal prescription. You should be registered with your own medical practitioner in order to seek treatment for yourself.

Best practice indicates that you should never prescribe for family or for people close to you. The people you prescribe for should be under your care in a professional context as patients.

Only in exceptional circumstances may you prescribe for family, friends or colleagues. The General Medical Council (2013) identifies these circumstances as:

♦ When no other prescriber is available to assess the clinical condition and to delay prescribing would put the patient's life or health at risk or cause intolerable pain
♦ The treatment is immediately necessary to save life, avoid serious deterioration in the patient's health or wellbeing or alleviate otherwise uncontrollable pain.

If this were to happen in practice and there was any questioning of your actions or any adverse outcomes experienced by the patient, then you would have to justify your actions to your employer, to the NMC and potentially in court. This could jeopardise your prescribing qualification and your professional registration, and is therefore best avoided.

Your choice of treatment should be based on the best available evidence and reached in agreement with your patient. As part of their promotional activities, pharmaceutical company drug representatives may provide inexpensive gifts such as pens. Personal gifts that influence prescribing practice are not permitted and it is specified in the Human Medicines Regulations (2012) by law that a prescriber may not solicit or accept a gift, advantage, benefit or hospitality that could influence their prescribing decisions. You must work within the NHS, your organisation and regulatory body code of conduct when interacting with the pharmaceutical industry (RPS 2016).

Record-keeping

Prescribing activity should occur at the time of the consultation or contact with the patient to ensure it is contemporary and reflective of the actual events. Only in exceptional circumstances should the documentation occur after the prescribing event and this should never exceed 24 hours.

Your prescribing record should evidence that you have communicated the prescribing activity and decision with the patient's primary healthcare practitioner, such as their GP. For inpatient care, this could be in the form of a discharge letter.

Prescribing for Children

Prescribing for children comes with its own risks. Medicines are more potent in use for children and therefore carry a higher risk of adverse outcomes, as responses to medicines may be different. You should only prescribe for children if this is within your scope of prescribing practice and you are clinically competent, experienced, skilled and knowledgeable to do so. You should also only prescribe for children with your employer's support and with indemnity insurance. This is unlikely to be required in traditional UK district nursing contexts where service provision is for adults only.

You should refer to national and local policy guidance and the BNF for children before prescribing for children.

Prescribing in Pregnancy

Prescribing in pregnancy and for breastfeeding women carries increased risk. This is because of the risk of medicines reaching the baby and having a toxic effect. You should only prescribe in pregnancy and for breastfeeding women if this is within your scope of prescribing practice and you are clinically competent, experienced, skilled and knowledgeable to do so. You should only prescribe for pregnant women with your employer's support and indemnity insurance to do so.

It is important to remember that you are never prescribing in isolation and that there are many sources of support available to you when you are making prescribing decisions in complex areas such as pregnancy. You can call on colleagues in specialist areas such as obstetrics to assess and treat the patient or to advise you on the best course of action, and colleagues in pharmacy will also support you. Your BNF will also offer a comprehensive guide. It is important to assess and consider the risk-benefit ratio of a prescribing decision in your practice, i.e. is it safer to prescribe or not prescribe? However, you must remember that you are accountable for all your decisions and omissions, and therefore if you are unsure, or if this is outside of your prescribing practice, you should refer on, document and be able to justify your actions.

Prescribing and Dispensing, Prescribing and Administration

Except in very exceptional circumstances, there should always be a separation of the prescribing of and the dispensing or administration of medicines. If in exceptional circumstances a prescriber is prescribing and dispensing, then a second competent person should be involved in the checking process. Should this happen, the clear arrangements need to be in place to ensure patient and prescriber safety, and robust audit processes need to be in place.

This is reflective of the prescribing and administration of medicines. This should only happen in exceptional circumstances and in the best interests of the patient; a second person should check the medicine before administration to verify it is correct.

Controlled Drugs

Independent nurse prescribers can prescribe any medicine from the BNF if this is within their scope of practice and competence (NICE 2019b). This also includes unlicensed medicines and controlled drugs schedules 2–5 where it is clinically indicated and within your scope of prescribing practice (RCN 2019). These controlled drugs extend to diamorphine hydrochloride, dipipanone or cocaine for treating organic disease or injury but NOT for treating addiction (Department of Health 2012a; NICE 2019a). Independent nurse prescribers are able to prescribe other drugs for addiction if it is within their scope of practice and competence (NICE 2019b).

As a nurse independent prescriber, you are able to requisition controlled drugs, and are authorised to possess, supply, offer to supply and administer the drugs you are able to prescribe within your scope of practice and competence (NICE 2019a). Please see the prescribing and dispensing and prescribing and administration information above.

Additionally, as a district nurse independent prescriber, it may be appropriate for you to compete controlled drug authorisation charts, e.g. for use in palliative care in the home environment. Independent nurse prescribers are able to prescribe, administer and give directions for controlled drugs schedule 2, 3 and 5, extending to diamorphine hydrochloride, dipipanone or cocaine for treating organic disease or injury but not for treating addiction (NICE 2019a). This means that you can lawfully complete a medicines authorisation chart for controlled drugs, in palliative or end-of-life care, if it is within your scope of practice and competence, and with your employers and local health service providers agreement. This identifies that qualified nurses who are competent and safe to do so may administer these drugs under your authorisation if these prerequisites are in place.

With the changes to the Misuse of Drugs Act (Department of Health 2012b), independent nurse prescribers can mix any controlled drugs listed in schedules 2 to 5 with other medicines for patients who require intravenous infusion (RCN 2019).

Following the Shipman Inquiry (Fourth Report 2006), there are legal requirements for schedule 2–3 controlled drugs and these are summarised in the BNF. Recommendations for the prescriptions of controlled drugs which are now legal requirements include (NICE 2016):

♦ The registration number of the prescriber will be included on controlled drug prescriptions
♦ Prescriptions for controlled drugs will be uniquely marked to identify them as controlled drug prescriptions
♦ Private prescriptions for controlled drugs will be similar to NHS prescriptions with a standard written request form
♦ The patient's NHS number and other patient-specific identifiers will be included on the prescription
♦ Prescriptions for controlled drugs (except schedule 5 controlled drugs) will be valid for only 28 days from issue. This can be extended in exceptional circumstances only if endorsed as such by the prescriber appropriately on the prescription.

When making decisions about prescribing controlled drugs, it is important to consider a number of factors:

♦ The risk-benefit ratio of a controlled drug's therapeutic effect versus risk of dependence or overdose
♦ If the patient is opioid naive
♦ The evidence base of your prescribing options and of your decision.

When you are prescribing controlled drugs, documentation is paramount:

♦ All prescribing decisions need to be recorded in the patient's notes
♦ You must communicate your prescribing decisions and intervention to the practitioners involved in and responsible for the care of the patient, such as the GP, community palliative care team and out-of-hours services
♦ Discuss, plan and document; review and follow-up.

♦ Clearly record any further instructions for other healthcare personnel (such as drug authorisation charts)
♦ Clearly document medicine instructions, such as when and how to take/administer the drug, including drug doses and frequency
♦ Consider and document and dose adjustments that may be required. This could be due to the likelihood of increased symptoms in progressive disease or due to reduced body mass index in cachexia.

Other best practice guidance includes(NICE 2016):

♦ When altering or reviewing controlled drug regimes, do so in line with local and national guidance and formularies. Seek advice from other clinicians when required.
♦ Use a recognised opioid dosing conversion tool when changing opioid in order to consider the total amount of opioid that will be systemically available.
♦ Follow your organisational policy and procedure and seek support when required.

NICE offers evidence-based guidelines on the safe use and management of controlled drugs; there is also useful comprehensive information on the BNF website to assist prescribers.

Evidence-based Prescribing

The act of prescribing is only one part of the decision-making process. Evidence-based prescribing is an approach to decision making, considering and applying the best available evidence in the treatment of your patients (Courtenay and Griffiths 2010). When drawing on evidence, district nurse independent prescribers should source national primary evidence in the first instance. If this is not available, then you can turn to local protocols or evidence for prescribing (NICE 2016). This will be relative to the context in which your patient is presenting, as evidence-based practice differs from primary to secondary care. For example, an elderly patient presenting with a cough and comorbidities may receive first-line antibiotics in primary care, but in hospital they may receive a chest x-ray and blood testing.

As an independent prescriber you need to ensure that your practice is evidence-based and you need to be aware of the current evidence supporting the use of each medicine within your scope of prescribing practice. You should only prescribe according to the best available evidence to ensure efficacy of treatment; to minimise risk, adverse drug reactions and interactions; and to ensure that the most appropriate medicine is chosen (RPS 2016).

As discussed previously in this chapter, prescribing needs to be appropriate as well as evidence-based, and patients must be involved in the prescribing decision and be able to make informed choices regarding their choices, where

---

Box 9.3 – Nurse prescribers' 'must do' list

♦ Be familiar with national sources of evidence, e.g. the National Institute for Health and Care Excellence (NICE), the British Thoracic Society (BTS) and the Scottish Intercollegiate Guidelines Network (SIGN).
♦ Be familiar with the national sources of evidence for the condition you are treating, what should and should not be used and the hierarchy of medicine use. NICE and the BNF are valuable information sources.
♦ Take an appropriate holistic assessment of the patient.
♦ Take into account the patient's wishes and choices.
♦ Prescribe the appropriate dose for the patient's age, weight, height and medical history.
♦ Prescribe the correct duration and frequency of the medicine.

(College of Paramedics 2018)

---

possible. This may not be possible where a patient lacks capacity to make decisions.

To aid safe and effective evidence-based prescribing, the College of Paramedics (2018) has developed a 'must do' list which is also applicable to district nursing prescribing practice. This is detailed in Box 9.3.

Conclusion

This chapter has highlighted how the legal and ethical principles you apply in your practice can be adapted to prescribing practice by independent district nurse prescribers. Ensuring that you apply these principles will promote safe and effective decision making in prescribing practice. A key factor is to ensure that you involve the patient in the prescribing decision-making process and take care to make contemporaneous and detailed records that reflect the consultation and identify the rationale of the prescribing decision. The patient's perspective should also be included in your documentation.

Another key consideration is to ensure that you prescribe in your scope of prescribing practice and refer on when you feel that there is a prescribing decision to be made outside of your scope of prescribing practice or competence. You must always have assessed the patient you are prescribing for and must never prescribe in order to fill a deficit in the availability of others' ability to prescribe in practice, e.g. if there is a lack of resourcing.

Always ensure an evidence-based approach to your prescribing practice, based on the most recent and available national evidence, and be prepared to justify your prescribing decision to others based on this.

Key Points of This Chapter

◆ There is clear guidance provided by the NMC, the RCN and NICE, which has a foundation in the legal system surrounding prescribing.
◆ Prescribers need to be cognisant of the ethical considerations when prescribing.
◆ There are many factors that require the consideration of the independent nurse prescriber, but ultimately you must only prescribe in the areas in which you are knowledgeable, competent, safe and skilled to do so.

References and Further Reading

Beauchamp, T. L. and Childress, J. F. (2013) *Principles of Biomedical Ethics.* 7th edn. New York: Oxford University Press.

British National Formulary (BNF) (2017) *The British National Formulary 72: September 2016–March 2017.* London: The BMJ Group.

British National Formulary (BNF) (2018) *The British National Formulary 75: March–September 2018.* London: The BMJ Group.

British National Formulary (BNF) (2019) *The British National Formulary 75: March–September 2019.* London: The BMJ Group.

College of Paramedics (2018) *Practice Guidance for Paramedic Independent and Supplementary Prescribers.* Bridgwater: College of Paramedics.

Courtenay, M. and Griffiths, M. (2010) *Independent and Supplementary Prescribing: An Essential Guide.* Cambridge: Cambridge University Press.

Department of Constitutional Affairs (2005) *Mental Capacity Act.* London: The Stationery Office.

Department of Health (1989) *Report for the Advisory Group on Nurse Prescribing (Crown Report).* London: Department of Health.

Department of Health (2006) *Safer Management of Controlled Drugs: The Government's Response to the Fourth Report of the Shipman Inquiry.* London: Department of Health.

Department of Health (2012a) Nurse and pharmacist independent prescribing changes announced. Available at: https://www.gov.uk/government/news/nurse-and-pharmacist-independent-prescribing-changes-announced (last accessed 20 June 2019).

Department of Health (2012b) *Misuse of Drugs Act.* London: The Stationery Office.

Dimond, B. (2015) *Legal Aspects of Nursing.* 7th edn. London: Pearson.

England, E. (2016). Paramedics and medicines: Legal considerations. *Journal of Paramedic Practice* 8(8): 408–415.

General Medical Council (GMC) (2013) Good practice in prescribing and managing medications and devices. Available at: https://www.gmc-uk.org/-/media/documents/prescribing-guidance_pdf-59055247.pdf (last accessed 20 June 2019).

Health Care Professions Council (HCPC) (2018) Medicines and prescribing. Available at: https://www.hcpc-uk.org/education-providers/updates/2018/medicines-and-prescribing-keeping-programmes-up-to-date/ (last accessed 26 February 2020).

HM Government (1968) *Medicines Act*. London: The Stationery Office.

HM Government (1971) *Misuse of Drugs Act*. London: The Stationery Office.

HM Government (2012) *Humans Medicines Regulations*. London: The Stationery Office.

Institute for Apprenticeship and Technical Education (2019) District nurse apprenticeship standard. Available at: https://instituteforapprenticeships.org/apprenticeship-standards/district-nurse/ (last accessed 13 May 2019).

Medicines and Healthcare products Regulatory Agency (MHRA) (2019) Medicines and Healthcare products Regulatory Agency. Available at: https://www.gov.uk/government/organisations/medicines-and-healthcare-products-regulatory-agency (last accessed 20 June 2019).

National Institute of Health and Care Excellence (NICE) (2014) Off-label or unlicensed use of medicines: Prescribers' responsibilities. Available at: https://www.gov.uk/drug-safety-update/off-label-or-unlicensed-use-of-medicines-prescribers-responsibilities (last accessed 28 November 2019).

National Institute of Health and Care Excellence (NICE) (2016) Recommendations for prescribing controlled drugs. Available at: https://www.nice.org.uk/guidance/NG46/chapter/Recommendations#prescribing-controlled-drugs 2019).

National Institute of Health and Care Excellence (NICE) (2019a) Non-medical prescribing. Available at: https://bnf.nice.org.uk/guidance/non-medical-prescribing.html accessed 20 June 2019).

National Institute of Health and Care Excellence (NICE) (2019b) Nurse and pharmacist independent prescribing changes announced. Available at: https://www.gov.uk/government/news/nurse-and-pharmacist-independent-prescribing-changes-announced (last accessed 20 June 2019).

NHS Education for Scotland (Nursing, Midwifery and Allied Health Professions) (2018) Out of hours unscheduled care: Advanced clinical practice portfolio. Available at: https://www.nes.scot.nhs.uk/media/463876/ooh_advanced_clinical_practice_portfolio.pdf (last accessed 10 August 2018).

NHS England (2014) *The Five Year Forward View*. London: NHS England.

NHS England (2019) *The NHS Long Term Plan*. London: NHS England.

Nurse Prescribers' Advisory Group (2017) *Nurse Prescribers' Formulary for Community Practitioners 2015–2017*. London: BNF.

Nursing and Midwifery Council (NMC) (2006) *Standards for Proficiency for Nurse and Midwife Prescribers*. London: NMC.

Nursing and Midwifery Council (NMC) (2018) *Realising Professionalism: Standards for Education and Training. Part 3: Standards for Prescribing Programmes*. London: NMC.

Nursing and Midwifery Council (NMC) (2019) Pre-2019 standards of prescribing practice. Available at: https://www.nmc.org.uk/standards/standards-for-post-registration/standards-for-prescribers/standards-of-proficiency-for-nurse-and-midwife-prescribers/ (last accessed 20 June 2019).

Royal College of Nursing (RCN) (2019) Non-medical prescribing. Available at: https://www.rcn.org.uk/get-help/rcn-advice/non-medical-prescribers (last accessed 20 June 2019).

Royal College of Nursing (RCN) (2019a). RCN Indemnity Scheme. Available at: https://www.rcn.org.uk/get-help/indemnity-scheme (last accessed 28 November 2019).

Royal Pharmaceutical Society (RPS) (2016) *A Competency Framework for all Prescribers.* London: RPS.

Chapter 10
Public Health and Prescribing

Hannah Ingram

In This Chapter

- ♦ Introduction
- ♦ Public health
- ♦ Public health outcomes framework
- ♦ Deprivation and health outcomes
- ♦ Public health and the prescribing role
- ♦ Antimicrobial resistance
- ♦ Antimicrobial stewardship and awareness
- ♦ Infection control
- ♦ Public health prescribing for older people
- ♦ Conclusion
- ♦ Key points of this chapter
- ♦ References and further reading.

Introduction

This chapter aims to give an overview of the public health aspects of prescribing practice for district nurses. It will outline the importance of incorporating a public health perspective into your prescribing practice in contemporary healthcare settings.

Public Health

Public health is defined as:

> 'The science and art of preventing disease, prolonging life and promoting health through the organised efforts of society' (Acheson 1988).

The objective of public health is to ensure that health inequalities are minimised and to ensure health and wellbeing for all. Public health focuses on the health and wellbeing of populations rather than of individuals (ISD Scotland 2010). As such, public health has been missing from the district nursing agenda for some time as the focus of care and service delivery has been reactive to the needs of individuals rather than communities and populations. Traditionally, public health work has been a separate speciality within UK healthcare contexts. Specialist public health roles within health and social care remain. Public health work has become common practice and examples are:

♦ Monitoring the health status of the population
♦ Identifying health needs
♦ Building programmes to reduce risk and screen for early signs of disease
♦ Preventing/controlling communicable diseases
♦ Developing policies to promote health.

However, with the increase in chronic disease, an ageing population with longer life expectancy and with finite resources available for health and social care, public health has become the business of every healthcare professional.

Public health initiatives are traditionally focused on prevention rather than cure, and as such district nurses have been advised that, as a reactive rather than proactive service, public health is not part of their remit. However, prevention rather than cure is a huge part of the district nursing role and that of district nurse independent prescribers. District nurses are a vital element of the NHS, who keep people well and out of hospital and who are able to deliver early interventions (Bhardwa 2015).

You will be well aware of the hospital avoidance agenda in contemporary healthcare policy. This is an excellent example of a public health concern of district nursing practice and of independent prescribing by district nurses. There has been an overall shift in healthcare policy to focus on the delivery of care and services in the primary care arena, with the focus on keeping people out of hospital and cared for at home, and district nurse prescribers have a fundamental role in facilitating this. This identifies that public health requires multi-level collaborative approaches to ensure success in meeting targets and reducing health inequalities (Nuttall 2008a).

Individual Public Health Approaches

The skills you have as a district nurse will be conducive with the contemporary approach to public health, with its socially determined positive concepts of health and where each individual patient interaction is the potential to promote and achieve public health issues (Naidoo and Earle 2007). Therefore, similarly, every prescribing interaction you have with an individual patient is an opportunity to promote health and address public health issues (Nuttall 2008a).

The pressures of contemporary healthcare, with reduced finances available for health and social care, ageing populations with more long-term conditions and a younger population that continues to make poorer lifestyle choices in Western society, mean there are increasing health needs. Public health policy is now incorporating an individual-based, as well as a population-based approach to care. Long-term diseases are closely linked to behavioural risk factors, and around 40% of the UK's disability adjusted life years lost can be attributed to obesity, alcohol, smoking and a sedentary lifestyle (NHS England 2018).

Think about:

What strategies do you employ in your practice that facilitate an individual-based public health approach?

An example of individual approaches to public health can be seen in the 'Making Every Contact Count' (MECC) initiative. MECC is an approach to behaviour change that utilises the interactions that health and social care providers have with people every day to encourage behaviour change that will have a positive impact on the health and wellbeing of individuals, communities and populations (NHS England 2018). It is possible for district nurse prescribers to adopt a MECC approach within their daily practice during consultations with patients to promote healthier behaviours. This approach can also be adopted for public health-related prescribing practice, and this will be discussed later.

Population-based Public Health Approaches

Population-based public health initiatives can be geographical, community, gender, age, disease or income-related, in order to define a group of people to be targeted for public health initiatives (Courtenay and Griffiths 2010).

The number of older people with substance misuse problems is increasing, with alcohol and illicit drugs among the top term risk factors for premature death and health problems, and mortality rates for illicit drug and alcohol-related deaths are higher for older people than for younger people (NHS England 2011). Alcohol misuse can also increase the likelihood of the misuse of prescription drugs (NHS England 2011).

The NHS reports that between 1992 and 2008, the highest alcohol-related death rates were recorded in men and women aged between 55 and 75 years old (NHS England 2011). Additionally, in 2008, 10% of older women reported drinking more than the recommended maximum recommended units and a fifth of older men reported drinking more than four units of alcohol on at least one day of the week. Among older people, the problem of alcohol misuse is often hidden.

Think about:

What organised efforts could be employed to address excess alcohol use in the UK?

The organised efforts of the UK in a public health approach to addressing excessive alcohol consumption in the UK, in an effort to reduce alcohol-related deaths and adverse outcomes and chronic disease, include:

♦ NICE guidelines – https://www.nice.org.uk/guidance/ph24
♦ Health services – treatment/advice/prevention strategies
♦ Police services – enforcing domestic violence / drink driving laws
♦ Local authorities – running education programmes and initiatives through health and social care services with the third sector, such as AGE UK
♦ National government – determining licensing laws and taxation.

The Public Health Outcomes Framework

The Public Health Outcomes Framework (PHOF) is a government initiative that helps public health officials identify trends and areas to target in order to improve health. It sets out a vision for public health in England and the desired outcomes. It identifies target areas for public health practice (Public Health England 2018). Some of these areas can be adopted and considered in your prescribing practice.

Public Health England (2018) identifies current public health areas for targeting in England. Those relevant to district nursing prescribing practice include:

♦ Tackling antibiotic resistance
♦ Reducing smoking and harmful drinking
♦ Reducing dementia risk
♦ Improving health and wellbeing
♦ Establishing prevention programmes (diabetes, falls etc.)
♦ Reducing the inequality in the uptake of screening
♦ Extending immunisation programmes.

It is possible to identify areas from this list that district nurses can contribute to in their daily prescribing consultations with patients using the MECC approach to public health. Health promotion and behaviour change through motivational interviewing approaches can address harmful drinking and smoking, as well as improving health and wellbeing.

Turn to **Chapter 11** for further information on motivational interviewing.

Promoting screening programmes and immunisation as part of your prescribing practice is an important part of your public health role. Screening programmes are available for a variety of age groups. Patients should be signposted to the appropriate programmes for their age and for the health conditions you are treating. For example, screening for bowel cancer is a priority target in older people and this should be promoted when undertaking prescribing interactions for altered bowel habits with older people. A large public health prescribing role in primary care is the annual flu vaccine programme. This may form part of your prescribing role, and this may also extend to the pneumonia vaccine. Additionally, this may include pandemic vaccination programmes as they arise in society, such as the bird flu pandemic.

As part of your prescribing role, when making prescribing decisions in practice with your patients, it is essential to consider the wider strategic initiatives and interventions you can access as part of your treatment plans to improve health and wellbeing. This can include referrals to prevention strategies, such as falls prevention or pulmonary rehabilitation programmes, where they are available. As a prescriber, you will find that you will develop a wide knowledge of services that would be of benefit to your patients but may not be available in your local area. As a district nurse and as a prescriber, it is important that you contribute to strategic initiatives in the consideration, planning and commissioning of services that will improve health and wellbeing in a public health approach to care.

Deprivation and Health Outcomes

In **Chapter 2**, we explored the wider determinants of health in relation to health assessment, consultation and prescribing. In looking at Dahlgren and Whitehead's (1991) model to promote equity in health, it can be established that greater deprivation and reduced health literacy can lead to poorer health outcomes. It is of value to reiterate here that as part of your prescribing consultations, it is important to explore any issues regarding deprivation, poverty or lack of health literacy. You are then able to use a public health approach to your prescribing practice, where you can address these by signposting where appropriate and identifying any areas for health screening in a preventative approach.

Greater deprivation can lead to poorer health outcomes (Buck and Maguire 2015), where preventative or reactive intervention may be required by district nurse prescribers. These include:

♦ Coronary heart disease
♦ Smoking
♦ Obesity
♦ Accidents
♦ Substance misuse.

When considering deprivation, poverty and treating people with low incomes, it is important to also consider the psychological impact that this has on individuals, as well as treating the physical health problems. In addition, in fiscal markets of healthcare provision and in times of austerity, services and welfare programmes are also cut. This can result in the more vulnerable people in society being adversely affected. Austerity, poverty and deprivation have a huge impact on mental health, which has the potential to cause problems for individuals and communities in the future (McGrath et al. 2015). In a holistic approach to prescribing practice, it is essential that you consider the mental health implications of prescribing decision making with patients.

Public Health and the Prescribing Role

Nuttall (2008a) discusses three domains of public health practice. These are explored here in relation to your practice as district nurse:

♦ Health improvement
♦ Services improvement
♦ Health protection.

Health improvement opportunities for public health from a prescribing perspective should arise from the consultation and assessment process. The key undertaking as a district nurse prescriber is to identify the public health opportunity in a patient interaction and act accordingly. This can be a challenge in practice due to time constraints, prioritisation of need and the breadth and depth of your scope of prescribing practice. It is important to remember that you do not have to address every issue at once with your patient. As a district nurse, you will most likely develop an ongoing relationship with your patients, and issues can be addressed at a later date or you can refer on to other practitioners in an integrated and collaborative approach. For health improvement in a public health context, any action is better than none (Nuttall 2008a).

Improving services can be undertaken by district nurse prescribers through participation in forums and through responding to relevant consultations to have an influence on policy for prescribing and for public health. In addition, you will need to remain up to date and competent in your prescribing practice to ensure an evidence-based approach. Your own professional reflection on and audit of your prescribing practice will aim to promote equity, cost-effectiveness and efficiency in your professional and prescribing practice and thus improve the service you deliver in a public health context (Nuttall 2008a).

Health protection for district nurse prescribers will include initiatives such as immunisations, e.g. flu and pneumonia vaccination programmes. Accidents such as falls are common in older people and can be related to a number of contributory factors such as alcohol and medications. Being able to identify and address risk in your professional and prescribing practice will help ensure the health protection of your patients and reduce any adverse outcomes (Nuttall 2008a).

As a district nurse independent prescriber, you may have perceived your public health role to be minimal in this context; however, on deeper reflection it is evident that the public health role of a prescriber is key.

Contemporary healthcare considerations and public health initiatives 'fit into' the district nurse prescribing role in a number of ways. These include:

♦ Duty to patients and society
♦ Policy regarding the use of antibiotics and vaccines
♦ Inappropriate use of medication, including over-use and under-use
♦ Inappropriate prescribing, over-prescribing and under-prescribing
♦ Access to healthcare provision and medicines.

Further generic guidance on public health professional practice is offered by the Faculty of Public Health in its Good Public Health Practice Framework (2016).

Think about:

What public health practices will you consider and incorporate into your daily prescribing practice as an independent district nurse prescriber?

Your public health prescribing role as a district nurse independent prescriber could include:

♦ De-prescribing
♦ Managing waste
♦ Reviewing repeat prescribing
♦ Antimicrobial stewardship
♦ Managing the misuse of medicines
♦ Managing polypharmacy – medicines optimisation
♦ Patient health education – MECC
♦ Leadership of teams and disseminating knowledge – professional expertise
♦ Evidence-based prescribing
♦ Cost-effective prescribing
♦ Use of and contribution to local formularies.

De-prescribing

De-prescribing is the process of stopping or reducing doses of medicine to manage polypharmacy and improve health outcomes. It requires careful consideration and should be done in a partnership approach with patients, utilising shared decision making. De-prescribing should form a part of your routine consultation with patients as a district nurse independent prescriber (BNF 2019).

Questions to consider when thinking about de-prescribing include the following:

♦ Is the drug still needed?
♦ Has the condition changed?
♦ Can the patient continue to benefit?

- ♦ Has the evidence changed?
- ♦ Have the guidelines changed (national or local)?
- ♦ Is the drug being used to treat an iatrogenic issue?
- ♦ What if any are the ethical issues concerning withholding the medicine?
- ♦ Would discontinuation cause problems?

Managing Waste

NICE identifies that due to polypharmacy caused by multi-morbidity, the average number of prescription items per person in the UK has risen from 13 to 19 (in 2013). NICE also identifies that adverse events, unplanned hospital admissions and poor outcomes can result from polypharmacy and from people not using their medicines correctly or as prescribed, which contributes to waste. A large amount of money is lost each year from the NHS due to the wasting of medicines. Issues to consider in your prescribing practice that may contribute to the waste of medicines are as follows:

- ♦ Patients recovering before their dispensed medicines have been taken
- ♦ Therapies being stopped or changed because of ineffectiveness or unwanted side effects
- ♦ Patients' conditions progressing so that new medicines are required
- ♦ Factors relating to repeat prescribing and dispensing processes, which may cause excessive volumes of medicines to be supplied, independently of any patient action
- ♦ Care system failures to support medicines taken by vulnerable individuals living in the community, who cannot independently adhere fully to their prescribed treatment regimes
- ♦ Medicines prescribed during a hospital stay being continued unnecessarily when the patient returns home
- ♦ Patients stockpiling 'just in case' medicines and reordering repeat medication that they do not need.

It is important to consider the effective use of medicines in your prescribing practice, with a view to any potential unnecessary waste that may be caused as a result of your prescribing decisions. In fiscal healthcare markets, sustainability and the need for cost-efficiency are paramount in prescribing practice.

Patient Health Education

The health literacy of patients and the opportunities for health behaviour change using MECC and motivational interviewing strategies have been discussed. This may not be limited to health promotion advice around health behaviour; it may also include informing patients about the best evidence available regarding the choices they may need to make about their health. Due to access to the internet, media sources and a plethora of information available, it can be a challenge for patients to reach decisions based on the best available evidence. It must also be remembered that some people, for a variety of reasons, may not have access to the wealth of electronic information and in your consultations this must be remembered if you are suggesting that your patient should 'find out more'.

Over-use and Misuse of Medicines

Contributing to the waste of medicines in contemporary healthcare is the over-use and misuse of medication. The irrational use of medicines is a major threat to health and leads to a waste of resources. This misuse or over-use of medicines accounts for half the global use of medicines (WHO 2012). As with non-adherence to medicine regimes, there can be unintentional and intentional over-use/misuse of medicines.

It can be a challenge for prescribers to identify where there is an over-use or misuse of medicines. There can be signs and symptoms displayed that may provide cues as to the over-use or misuse of medicines, and as a prescriber it is important to be able to recognise these and address them with your patients. These include the following:

♦ Losing medication so that more prescriptions are required – this can become a pattern
♦ Seeking prescriptions from various healthcare professionals or practices
♦ Requesting a specific drug, as others do not work
♦ Stealing or forging prescriptions
♦ Appearing intoxicated or sedated or experiencing withdrawal symptoms
♦ Mood swings or hostility
♦ Increase or decrease in sleep.

If you are unsure in relation to the identification of the over-use or misuse of medicines in your patients within your prescribing practice, seek support from your colleagues in the management of such challenges.

Non-intentional Over-use/Misuse

One of the most common forms of unintentional over-use or misuse of medicines involves paracetamol. Patients may be unaware of the paracetamol content of cough and cold medicines and may take these in addition to paracetamol doses for a prolonged duration, which can have fatal consequences. It is imperative that patients are counselled on the use of paracetamol-containing medicines as part of your prescribing practice.

Antimicrobial Resistance

The main cause of concern in contemporary prescribing practice for district nurses with over-prescribing is that of antibiotics.

The term 'antimicrobial' refers not only to antibacterial medicines such as antibiotics but also to antimicrobials, antiprotozoals, antivirals and antifungals medicines (Courtenay and Griffiths 2010). There has been a developing resistance to antibiotic therapy since 1969. This problem is developing and there is now multi-resistance, with strains of bacteria becoming resistant to two or more unrelated antimicrobials. A high percentage of hospital-acquired infections (HAIs) are caused by highly resistant bacteria such as methicillin-resistant Staphylococcus aureus (MRSA) or multi-drug gram-negative bacteria.

The consequences of such resistance are that infections are more difficult to treat, drugs become more expensive in the quest to treat the infections and the infections remain contagious (Courtenay and Griffiths 2010). Increased hospital stays are associated with HAIs, which have known adverse effects for patients and result in more costs for already-stretched resources. In addition to financial costs, there is the human cost of increased mortality rate, in particular from MRSA and Clostridium difficile. NHS England (2014) estimates that these 'superbugs' will cause more deaths in the UK than cancer by 2050.

Antimicrobial Stewardship and Awareness

The focus of contemporary health policy in terms of antimicrobial stewardship is on antibacterial medicines, such as antibiotics. There is also growing resistance to antifungal drugs and antiviral medication used in the treatment of Human Immunodeficiency Virus (HIV) and influenza (Courtenay and Griffiths 2010).

In response to the growing concern of antimicrobial resistance, NHS England and Public Health England (2015) have launched collaborative awareness campaigns for health professionals and the public to highlight the problem and promote action. The key messages from Public Health England (2019) for prescribers in the effective delivery of antimicrobial stewardship are summarised in **Box 10.1**.

The considerations listed in **Box 10.1** are essential for your prescribing practice and should be reviewed in every consultation where an antimicrobial prescription is being considered.

Local and national guidelines and formularies will guide you on the correct antimicrobial prescription for the presenting complaint, which will be

Box 10.1 – Key messages for effective delivery of antimicrobial stewardship

- Right drug, at the right dose, at the right time, for the right duration
- Avoid unnecessary lengthy durations of antibiotic treatment
- Avoid inappropriate use of broad-spectrum antibiotics
- Communication is key – ensure patients have the right information
- Consider delayed prescriptions where appropriate.

based on the best available evidence. Each NHS organisation will have an evidence-based guide and formulary for the prescribing of antibacterial medicines due to increased resistance. These will also alert you as the prescriber to the correct dose, duration and formulation to treat the presenting complaint. Microbiology can come in useful where there appears to be no improvement in the condition, or formularies offer second-line choices if the patient is unable to use the preferred antimicrobial for any reason, such as allergy or drug interaction. For example, trimethoprim cannot be used with phenytoin (BNF 2019).

Patient counselling in the use of antimicrobials is essential in prescribing practice. Not only does this promote adherence, so that the patient will receive the optimal outcomes from their therapy, but education and counselling the patient will also ensure the effective use of the medicine. It is hoped that this will prevent further prescriptions being required and will prevent the development of any resistance. It is imperative that patients are educated in the use of antimicrobials, as taking these inappropriately or incorrectly can have potentially serious adverse outcomes. Patients must use the correct dosage and complete the course of antibacterial medicines. Patients should be advised not to share antibiotics or to use other people's antibiotics; this is not appropriate and will increase the risk of resistance and potential side effects.

When it is appropriate to prescribe antimicrobials as an independent district nurse prescriber, this action should be taken in partnership with your patient. However, when the clinical symptoms are not indicative of a bacterial infection, antibiotics should not be prescribed if they are not indicated. Alternative advice should be given to the patient, or patients should be directed to other healthcare professionals for advice, such as a community pharmacist.

Public Health England (2017) have provided a very useful toolkit for prescribers to help focus their practice on antimicrobial stewardship, as has the Royal College of General Practitioners (RCGP 2018).

Infection Control

Effective infection control procedures will reduce the spread of infection and the need for antimicrobials. Good infection control and prudent antimicrobial use by district nurse prescribers will ensure safe and effective care.

Public Health Prescribing for Older People

Increasing longevity in life expectancy has resulted in an ageing population. Life expectancy is estimated at 15.8 years at 60, a rise from 14.3 years in 2000 (WHO 2018). Internationally, people are living longer and healthier lives (Buck et al. 2015). Despite the international increase in life expectancy, this has stalled in the UK and there remains a large population of older people in the

UK who are living with ill health and long-term conditions requiring care (Buck et al. 2018; Coulter et al. 2013).

This means that the needs of older people are being met through a system that was not designed, has not evolved and is not equipped to meet the complex needs of older people who may be experiencing multiple long-term conditions. The current NHS was designed on a single disease and medical model (Buck et al. 2018; Humphries et al. 2016; Oliver et al. 2014), with minimal investment in older people's services (Ham 2014). This can leave older people marginalised, with a lack of opportunity to meet their own healthcare needs or access resources. This poses a problem for district nurse prescribers, as such limitations in older people's care will have an influence on prescribing decisions. As a district nurse prescriber, it is important that such inequalities and limitations to older people's care are addressed and reduced in a public health approach (Nuttall 2008b).

Inequalities for Older People

Access to Health Services
Inequalities for older people include the access to health services. Many older people rely on family and carers to provide assistance in accessing health and social care services; a lack of social support can negate access to services which will enhance care. Additionally, older people who are housebound may not be able to access services outside of their homes, leaving them at a disadvantage in terms of treatments and interventions. As a district nurse prescriber, it is your public health role to work in partnership with patients to identify how these inequalities may be reduced.

Social Isolation
A lack of contact with others results in social isolation and poor health outcomes. Part of the public health role of an independent prescriber is to assess for social isolation in older people to address how this can be alleviated in partnership with the patient in a holistic approach to prescribing practice.

Age Discrimination
Age discrimination still exists for older people. Contemporary society can treat older people unfairly, with preconceived ideas and prejudices of life after 65 years. One out of five adults experiences ageism in healthcare settings in America (Senior Living 2019). Stereotyping of older people is prevalent across society and manifests in preconceptions such as (Sage Minder 2019):

♦ Cannot remember things
♦ Cannot see or hear well
♦ Must be physically frail or weak
♦ Are inflexible and stubborn
♦ Cannot learn new things
♦ Must be interested in retiring
♦ Must not be capable of using technology

Clearly, these generalisations and stereotypes are unacceptable and must be addressed. As a district nurse prescriber, it is paramount that you address such issues when these are identified in your professional practice, but also that your prescribing decisions are based on evidence and are individual to the patient you are interacting with to ensure a patient-centred approach to safe and effective prescribing practice.

Housing

Housing is linked to the ability of people to achieve health and wellbeing (DoH 2006). As a district nurse you will be prescribing within the context of a patient's own home. This will give you a unique opportunity to assess and address the housing situation of your patients. From a public health and prescribing perspective, you need to also consider the concept of home for the older person and how this will influence prescribing decisions. For example, some older people may be averse to the medicalisation of their home environment with equipment and medication. A person-centred approach to prescribing decisions is essential, with the person being central to decision making.

There are some public health issues that affect older people specifically and which need to be considered by district nurse prescribers

Accidents

Accidents are a public health issue for older people. This includes falls. Falls are a serious problem for older people, as they have the highest risk of falling. Thirty per cent of people over 65 years and 50% of people over the age of 80 fall at least once a year. Falls result in pain, injury, disability, loss of confidence and independence, anxiety and death. Falls and the result of falls also affect carers and family members and have a cost to the NHS of £2.3 billion per year (NICE 2013). The risk of falls can be due to environmental, medication, ill health or ageing factors. As a district nurse independent prescriber, you should be able to identify and address any contributory factors to the risk of falls. Part of your consultation and assessment of older people should include a falls history, and contributory factors such as sensory impairment, alcohol use, incontinence, mobility, multiple pathologies and environmental hazards (Nuttall 2008b).

Wellbeing

Lifestyle advice is as appropriate for older people as it is for younger population groups. Positive health behaviours such as exercise, healthy eating and smoking cessation will improve health outcomes and wellbeing at any stage in the lifecycle (Nuttall 2008b). Initiatives such as MECC and motivational interviewing are key for addressing such interventions.

It is important to also consider that the focus of contemporary healthcare policy of living well in older age or of active ageing can add pressure to older people to be 'well' when they are experiencing ill health and disease. This can result in patients not reporting some problems to district nurses as they do not wish to be seen as a burden or as not coping with ill health. This highlights the need for individual person-centred assessment and decision making to ensure holistic needs are addressed and safe and effective prescribing practice occurs.

Admission Avoidance

The cost of multiple long-term conditions in conjunction with a healthcare system that is under-resourced and ill-equipped to deal with increasing demand has led to healthcare policy directives being focused on care in the community and avoidance of unnecessary hospital admissions. As prescribers, district nurses are paramount in facilitating admission avoidance and early discharge from acute services, and in working with patients, families and carers to avoid crisis or ill health and to self-manage long-term conditions in the community.

As a district nurse prescriber, it is essential to consider that sometimes people will need to attend hospital due to the nature of their ill health and you must work as part of a wider team to ensure that the patient receives the right care, at the right time, in the right place. It is important not to feel pressured as a prescriber to keep people out of hospital when this is not in their best interests.

Additionally, the focus on self-care is not always appropriate for all older people; some, due to the nature of their ill health and disease pathologies, may find that being able to self-care is not something they want or are able to facilitate. As a district nurse prescriber, working in partnership with patients and making shared decisions will ensure that person-centred safe and effective prescribing practice occurs.

Conclusion

This chapter has discussed concepts of public health in UK healthcare practice. The application of a public health perspective to district nurse prescribing and how this can be implemented in practice has been discussed, using several examples. Some of the complexities of prescribing in a public health context for older people have been considered. The importance of antimicrobial stewardship as an independent prescriber has been highlighted in response to public health issues of antimicrobial resistance.

Key Points of This Chapter

- ◆ The notion of public health has been explored in relation to independent prescribing by district nurses.
- ◆ Public health interventions, assessment of health risk and health promotion are part of the role of the district nurse prescriber.
- ◆ Older people have specific public health needs that need to be considered by district nurse prescribers.
- ◆ Antimicrobial stewardship is a serious public health issue and the district nurse prescriber needs to be fully aware of the most current advice and where to access relevant 'toolkits'.

References and Further Reading

Academy of Medical Sciences (2016) *Improving the Health of the Public by 2040.* London: Academy of Medical Sciences.

Acheson, E. D. (1988) *Public Health in England: Report of the Committee of Inquiry into the Future Development of the Public Health Function.* London: Department of Health.

Bhardwa, S. (2015) District nurses are a key component in public health. *Independent Nurse.* Available at: http://www.independentnurse.co.uk/news/district-nurses-key-component-in-public-health/75121/ (last accessed 7 August 2019).

British National Formulary (BNF) (2017) *The British National Formulary 74, September 2017–March 2018.* London: BMJ Group.

British National Formulary (BNF) (2019) *The British National Formulary 77, March–September 2019.* London: BMJ Group.

Buck, D. and Maguire, D. (2015) *Inequalities in Life Expectancy, Changes over Time and Implications for Policy.* London: The King's Fund.

Coulter, A., Roberts, S. and Dixon, A. (2013) *Delivering Better Services for People with Long Term Conditions. Building the House of Care.* London: The King's Fund.

Courtenay, M. and Griffiths, M. (2010) *Independent and Supplementary Prescribing: An Essential Guide.* 2nd edn. Cambridge: Cambridge University Press.

Dahlgren, G. and Whitehead, M. (1991) *Policies and Strategies to Promote Social Equity in Health.* Stockholm: Institute of Future Studies.

Department of Health (DoH) (2006) *Our Health, Our Care, Our Say. A New Direction for Community Services.* London: Department of Health.

Earle, S. and J. Naidoo. (2007) 'Who promotes public health?' In S. Earle, C. Lloyd, M. Sidell and S. Spurr (eds), *Theory and Research in Promoting Public Health.* London: Sage: 101–128.

Faculty of Public Health (2016) Good Public Health Practice Framework. Available at: https://www.fph.org.uk/media/1304/good-public-health-practice-framework_-2016_final.pdf (last accessed 28 November 2019).

Ham, C. (2014) *Priorities for the Next Government.* London: The King's Fund.

Humphries, R., Thorlby, R., Holder, H. et al. (2016) *Social Care for Older People. Home Truths.* London: The King's Fund.

ISD Scotland (2010) Public health. Available at: https://www.isdscotland.org/Health-Topics/Public-Health/ (last accessed 7 August 2019).

McGrath, L., Griffin, V. and Mundy, E. (2015) *The Psychological Impact of Austerity: A Briefing Paper.* London: Psychologists against Austerity.

National Institute for Health and Clinical Excellence (NICE) (2013) Falls in older people; assessing risk and prevention. London: NICE. Available at: https://www.nice.org.uk/guidance/cg161/ (last accessed 7 August 2019).

National Institute for Health and Clinical Excellence (NICE) (2015) *Antimicrobial Stewardship: Systems and Processes for Effective Antimicrobial Medicine Use.* London: NICE.

NHS England (2011) Elderly need drug and alcohol support. Available at: https://www.nhs.uk/news/older-people/elderly-need-alcohol-and-drug-support/ (last accessed 28 November 2019).

NHS England (2014) *Review on Antimicrobial Resistance.* London: NHS England.

NHS England (2018) Making every contact count. Available at: http://www.makingeverycontactcount (last accessed 28 November 2019).

NHS England and Public Health England (2015) Patient Safety Alert. Addressing antimicrobial resistance through and implementation of an antimicrobial stewardship programme. Available at: https://www.england.nhs.uk/wp-content/uploads/2015/08/psa-amr-stewardship-prog.pdf (last accessed 28 November 2019).

Nuttall, D. (2008a) Introducing public health to prescribing practice. *Nurse Prescribing* 6(7): 299–304.

Nuttall, D. (2008b) Older people, prescribing and public health. *Nurse Prescribing* 6(8): 357–361.

Office for National Statistics (2013) *Alcohol-Related Deaths, United Kingdom.* London: Office for National Statistics.

Oliver, D., Foot, C. and Humphries, R. (2014) *Making Our Health Care Systems Fit for an Ageing Population.* London: The King's Fund.

Public Health England (2018) Public health outcomes framework. Available at: https://www.fingertips.phe.org.uk/profile/public-health-outcomes-framework (last accessed 28 November 2019).

Public Health England (2019) Antibiotic awareness: Key messages. Available at: https://assets.publishing.service.gov.uk/government/uploads/system/uploads/attachment_data/file/836392/Antibiotic_Awareness_Key_messages_2019.pdf (last accessed 28 November 2019).

Royal College of General Practitioners (RCGP) (2018) TARGET antibiotic toolkit. Available at: http://www.rcgp.org.uk/clinical-and-research/resources/toolkits/amr/target-antibiotic-toolkit.aspx (last accessed 26 February 2020).

Sage Minder (2019) Ageism and the elderly. Available at: https://www.sageminder.com/SeniorHealth/Issues/AgeDiscrimination.aspx (last accessed 7 August 2019).

Senior Living (2019) How ageism in healthcare is affecting society. Available at: https://www.seniorliving.org/health/ageism/ (last accessed 7 August 2019).

Turner, G. M., Calvert, M., Feltham, M. G. et al. (2016) Under-prescribing of prevention drugs and primary prevention of stroke and transient ischaemic attack in the UK general practice: A retrospective analysis. *PHOS Medicine*. DOI: 10.1371/journal.pmed.1002169.

World Health Organization (WHO) (2012) *The Pursuit of Responsible Use of Medicines: Sharing and Learning from Country Experiences*. Geneva: World Health Organization.

World Health Organization (WHO) (2018) Global health observatory data repository. Life expectancy and healthy life expectancy. Available at: http://apps.who.int/gho/data/view.main-wpro.SDG2016LEXREGv?lang=en (last accessed 7 December 2018).

Chapter 11
Medicines Optimisation
Jennifer Gorman and Hannah Ingram

Introduction

Medicines are the most widely used therapeutic interventions in healthcare (RPS 2013). They are used to prevent illness, maintain health, manage chronic conditions and cure disease. Despite this, medicines are often not used as prescribed, meaning that patients may not be getting the best therapeutic outcomes from their treatment. In this chapter, we will consider some of the reasons why this is happening and how as prescribers you can support patients in optimising the outcomes from their medicines.

What is Medicines Optimisation?

Medicines optimisation is defined in NICE (2016) QS 120: Medicines Optimisation as 'a person-centred approach to safe and effective medicines use, to ensure people obtain the best possible outcomes from their medicines'. Before medicines optimisation came into use, the term 'medicines management' was often used in prescribing and healthcare practice. Medicines management focused more on processes around how medicines were used and was not predominantly patient-centred. The recognition that patient outcomes rely on patient participation and collaboration in the prescribing process led to this change in focus. The key paper from the Royal Pharmaceutical Society (RPS) (2013) describes medicines optimisation as a step change needed to address the all-too-common problem of medicines use being sub-optimal. It identifies four guiding principles to support the process of medicines optimisation in practice, which aim to improve patient outcomes, as outlined in Box 11.1.

As a prescriber, you will have a key role to play in supporting this process. Within the consultation you will need to understand the patient's experience and integrate this within the prescribing process. You will need to be able to discuss with them the evidence base behind treatment choices and make sure medicines use is as safe as possible. Crucially, this should be part of your routine practice. These four principles embed patient-centred, evidence-based, safe and effective prescribing practice.

To achieve this way of working, the patient's beliefs and experiences are key in the prescribing process, meaning healthcare professionals of all disciplines must work in partnership with their patients and other healthcare professionals. The goal of this collaboration is to:

♦ Improve patient outcomes
♦ Support patients to take their medicines correctly
♦ Avoid prescribing and taking of unnecessary medicines
♦ Reduce wastage of medicines
♦ Improve medicines safety.

Box 11.1 – RPS (2013) four guiding principles of medicines optimisation

1. Aim to understand the patient's experience
2. Evidence-based choice of medicines
3. Ensure medicines use is as safe as possible
4. Make medicines optimisation part of routine practice

Think about:

♦ What do you need in order to undertake effective medicines optimisation in your prescribing practice?
♦ What services do you know of that you can signpost patients to that support medicines optimisation?

Communication and Consultation Skills

Clear, concise, effective communication is essential in all aspects of prescribing practice and is key to supporting patients in optimising their medicines use. Eliciting from the patients their beliefs and experiences and then effectively relaying complex information to them around choices of medicines requires a high level of clinical communication skill.

Key Communication Activities Within the Consultation:

♦ Eliciting the patient's beliefs and experiences
♦ Discussing the evidence base behind treatment options
♦ Checking understanding of the prescribed regimen
♦ Monitoring of efficacy of the medicines.

Following a consultation, you will also need to document clearly what prescribing decisions have been made and give a rationale. This supports the ethos of medicines optimisation being a multidisciplinary activity, as clear documentation will allow other care providers to identify what options have been rejected and why, in order to inform future decision making.

You may wish to use some kind of model to support you as you develop your consultation skills in your new role of prescriber. Some clinicians do not like communication frameworks as they feel they can result in a consultation that appears to follow a tick-box approach. Conversely, others find it a supportive approach whilst they are developing in their role, in the knowledge that it may not fit every type of clinical interaction. Below, some of the most well-known models are briefly described, many of which include elements of ensuring sufficient attention is paid to a patient-centred approach. The reason for including these brief descriptions is to help you decide if one model fits with your way of working more intuitively. This means that if you are interested in finding out more about a particular model in more detail, you can use the references provided at the end of the chapter to do so.

ICE: Ideas, Concerns and Expectations

The importance of gathering information about the patient's ideas, concerns and expectations in terms of both diagnosis and management of disease is a common theme in clinical communication literature (Deveugele et al. 2005; Matthys et al. 2009; Pendleton 1984; Silverman et al. 2013). ICE as a simple mnemonic can be a useful aide memoire to ensure your consultation includes a focus on the patient's beliefs and needs. For more on the impact of ICE on prescribing, see Matthys et al. (2009).

Pendleton

This model was published as part of *The Consultation – An Approach to Learning and Teaching* (Pendleton 1984). The model features seven patient-centred tasks, which consist of defining the patient's agenda, considering other problems, choosing a management plan, achieving a shared understanding, using time and resources appropriately, and establishing and maintaining a relationship with the patient.

Neighbour

Neighbour (1987) published a five-step model in *The Inner Consultation*. This model focuses on key activities to be undertaken in the consultation.

The five steps of the Neighbour model are:

1. **Connecting:** This includes developing a working relationship with a patient, gathering information, along with developing a rapport
2. **Summarising:** This includes summarising the information into a diagnosis and creating a plan with the patient
3. **Handover:** This includes explaining and agreeing with the patient the management plan as well as handing responsibility for some elements back to the patient
4. **Safety-netting:** This includes making sure the patient knows what to do if things don't work out as planned and creating a contingency plan
5. **Housekeeping:** This includes making time to ensure that the clinician is able to be efficient and effective. It acknowledges that prescribers are human, and this is an important element that needs to be remembered and addressed. This means taking steps to address issues such as fatigue, stress or the effect of emotions.

Calgary-Cambridge Model

This is a popular framework used in medical education. It was first published in 1998, but has been updated and revised by the authors several times, most recently in 2013. It covers everything from the moment you say hello to the patient to the moment you say goodbye. It follows a five-step model, with two further elements that are threaded through the consultation: building a rapport and providing structure. This is shown in **Figure 11.1**.

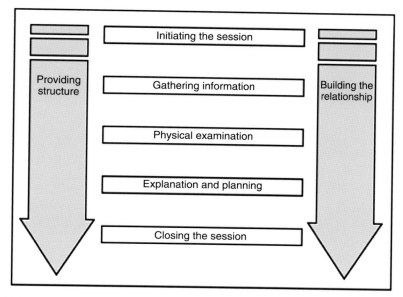

Figure 11.1 – The Calgary-Cambridge basic framework of structuring a medical interview

Source: Silverman et al. (2013). Reproduced with permission.

Think about:

Developing your own consultation style takes time and practice. While going through your NMP training:

♦ Watch how your prescribing supervisor does their consultations. Think about what works well, as well as anything you might do differently.

♦ Is there anything you can try in your own consultations that might improve how you consult with patients?

♦ Talking about risk can be challenging but it is an important part of medicines optimisation. If you see a consultation where the risk of taking or not taking a medicine is discussed, how is the risk explained and does the patient understand it?

Collaboration and Sharing Information

As already seen in the models above, collaboration with the patient is an essential part of optimising medicines use. It is not only the patient that you need to collaborate with, however. Collaboration with colleagues across services, especially when there has been a transfer in care, is paramount to ensuring there are no errors in medicine. This can be challenging for new prescribers. If in a transfer of care – for example, on hospital discharge – you identify a prescribing error, it can be difficult as a new prescriber to challenge the prescribing practice of another healthcare professional. However, this is essential to do, not only as a professional registrant but also for patient safety. This can be done in a collegiate and reflective manner to ensure there is learning and an improvement in practice. Likewise, if your prescribing practice is challenged, to have identified your rationale for your decision in the patient's records will help you reflect on why and how you reached the decision you did so that you can reflectively critique this should you be required to do so. A key part of collaborative working is also ensuring that all records about the patient are kept up to date. Some examples that link to medicines optimisation are:

- ♦ Documenting any changes to medication regimens, such as when medicines have been started or stopped. A reason for this decision should also be documented.
- ♦ Allergies/ADRs should always be recorded, along with the nature and severity of the reaction
- ♦ Any information that has been given to the patient and the carer/family regarding medicines and their use
- ♦ Any information on when medicines should be reviewed.

The key things to consider are whether you have provided enough information to ensure that another prescriber would be able to make an informed prescribing decision based on this? Also, there are strict regulations on storing of data and sharing of personal information – are you following best practice in relation to the General Data Protection Regulation (GDPR)?

Turn to **Chapter 10** to explore various means of improving your reflective practice.

Using Evidence-based Medicine to Support Medicines Optimisation

One of the RPS' (2015) guiding principles is using evidence-based medicine to underpin prescribing decisions. To achieve this, you will be expected to have a therapeutic knowledge of medicines use, plus their indications, place in therapy and any safety issues. While this knowledge will not be in-depth for every medicine in the British National Formulary (BNF), it should be for the medicines within your scope of prescribing practice. Also, if you are prescribing for a patient on medicines that you are not familiar with, a key skill is to know where to go to find information to make sure your prescribing is safe and effective. The BNF is the resource that most people will commonly go to for information about specific drugs. However, there are also a whole range of useful general prescribing information that people often miss. For example, there are sections dedicated to drug interactions, prescription writing and prescribing in renal and liver disease. To ensure medicines use is safe and effective, you should also be familiar with local and national guidelines related to your scope of practice. Local areas usually provide online access to the local drug formulary and relevant guidance; make sure you know how to access yours. You can also access information about drugs used in managing specific therapeutic areas via the NICE Clinical Knowledge Summaries (CKS), which are available at: https://cks.nice.org.uk/#?char=A. For complex prescribing problems, it is important to know your limitations and it may be necessary to seek assistance from, or refer the patient to, another healthcare professional.

Turn to **Chapters 4** and **5** for more detailed information on pharmacology and prescribing in special groups.

Turn to **Chapter 7** for more detailed information on evidence-based medicines and prescribing using local formularies and clinical guidelines.

Think about:

Do you know where to access relevant and up-to-date local and national guidance to support medicines optimisation in your prescribing practice?

The Role of Medicines Management

Although medicines optimisation takes a patient-centred approach, this does not mean that the concept of medicines management has no place. In this section, we will consider some of the ways in which the more process-based element of medicines management can affect how patients access and use medicine.

A patient may intentionally not be adherent with their medication due to concerns about taking the drug, or due to their perception of whether they actually need it (Nunes et al. 2009). However, it may also be due to a more practical issue around the supply of that medicine. For example, patients sometimes struggle with remembering to order their medicines and run out. It may be that supporting the patient, or their families/carers, to order medicines online could help resolve this problem.

When prescribing, you should also take time to become familiar with whether there are any services that tie in with the medicines you are prescribing. Depending on commissioning by your CCG, there may be local arrangements in how patients can access medicines that are relevant to your practice. For example, some areas have agreements with local pharmacies that allow urgent access to end-of-life care drugs for palliative patients. There are also various arrangements on how patients can access repeat medicines if they find they have run out during the out-of-hours period, usually via a referral to a pharmacy by NHS 111.

In **Chapter 7** we looked at the financial constraints that we are faced with working within the NHS. Another way you can contribute to cost-effective prescribing is by working within systems for managing medicines and reducing waste. For example, if a patient is started on a new drug, only supply a small quantity initially to check for the efficacy and tolerability of the drug. Make sure that medicines are reviewed regularly and taken off repeat prescription when they have been stopped. This may seem obvious, but the amount of medicines wasted shows that there is still work to be done to implement these basic changes.

Medicines Reconciliation

Medicines reconciliation forms a key role in underpinning medicines optimisation, particularly around the high-risk time when a transfer of care occurs. This process can be defined as 'the process of identifying an accurate list of a person's current medicines and comparing it with the current list in use' (NICE 2016). It is only through doing this that discrepancies or changes can be identified. This has a huge role to play in ensuring medicines are used safely and effectively and is why such an emphasis is placed on this activity. Medicines reconciliation involves obtaining an accurate and contemporaneous list of the medicines that the patient is actually using. This can reduce unintentional prescribing errors, which have been found to be a source of patient harm. Studies have found that more than 40% of medication errors are believed to result from inadequate medicines reconciliation during admission, transfer and discharge of patients (SPS 2017). Of these identified errors, approximately 20% are believed to result in patient harm.

One important element that is often overlooked during medicines reconciliation is the use of over-the-counter (OTC) medicines and complementary therapies. Another is that patients might neglect to tell the clinician things they do not perceive as relevant. Real-life examples are given below. You can see from this list that not knowing about these could have serious consequences. One example is from a patient who presented with a DVT. It was not identified that she had been taking an oral contraceptive pill for several days, despite the fact that due to their prothrombotic properties they are contraindicated. This patient did not see the pill as a 'proper medicine' despite the fact that it is a prescription only medicine (POM). Specific questioning is needed to ensure that these are not missed – see below for questions that can be incorporated into routine practice.

Real-life examples of treatments patients have not disclosed initially in medicines reconciliation because they did not perceive them as relevant:

♦ The contraceptive pill
♦ St John's Wort
♦ Ibuprofen bought OTC
♦ Chemotherapy.

When Should Medicines Reconciliation Take Place?

Medicines reconciliation should occur whenever patients move between care settings. The timescales vary between primary and secondary care, and are given below (NICE 2015):

♦ When a person moves from one care setting to another for acute care, e.g. into hospital, it should take place within 24 hours (or sooner if clinically necessary).
♦ In primary care, medicines reconciliation should take place for all people who have been discharged from hospital or another care setting as soon as is practically possible, before a prescription or new supply of medicines is issued and within one week of the GP practice receiving the information.

NICE (2015) considers medicines reconciliation to be a skilled task and that it should be undertaken by staff who are trained and competent healthcare professionals. As a prescriber, you should certainly be competent in conducting thorough medicines reconciliations.

The 3Cs Approach to Medicines Reconciliation

The 3Cs mnemonic included in the Specialist Pharmacy Service (2017) document on improving the quality of medicines reconciliation can help you remember the steps in this process:

1. **Collecting** – collect information about what medicines the patient is prescribed and what medicines they are currently taking, as well as other information about the patient's experience of using medicines e.g. allergies, side effects, any physical problems using medication (such as dexterity problems when using inhalers). This information will be collected from a range of sources. Ideally, the patient should always be involved as a primary source of information. If not, then a family member or carer may be used. Secondary sources could include medicines in the home, repeat prescription order forms, the Summary Care Record (SCR) and Medicines Administration Record (MAR) charts.

2. **Checking** – this step involves checking whether the information collected about the medicines use matches the records you have about what the patient is supposedly prescribed.
3. **Communicating** – this step involves discussing with the patient any anomalies you have found and deciding with them how to resolve these. You will then document this to ensure that the patient records are up to date for the next person who is involved in the patient's care.

Key Points to Remember When Doing Medicines Reconciliation:

♦ Always check to see if the patient is taking anything OTC or using complementary therapies
♦ Do not rely on repeat prescription request forms as they only tell you what is prescribed, not what the patient is actually taking
♦ Use at least two sources of information where possible, e.g. the patient and a GP repeat request
♦ If using a blister pack/dossette box, remember to check for any other medicines that can't go in the box e.g. warfarin, insulin, antibiotics, eye drops, inhalers or weekly medications
♦ Involve patients and family members/carers where appropriate to find out if the patient is taking the medicines as prescribed. If they are not, find out what they are actually doing and if possible why they are unable/unwilling to take them
♦ Ensure any discrepancies are documented, along with the reason, e.g. patient suffered side effect or medicine stopped by consultant at last hospital visit

---

Questions you may want to ask as part of the medicines reconciliation process:

♦ Does anybody help you with your medicines?
♦ Can you tell me about the medicines that you use every day?
♦ Are there any medicines that have been started, stopped or changed recently?
♦ Can you tell me about any problems you have had taking any medicines?
♦ Have you taken any courses of antibiotics recently?
♦ Do you use any medicines that you buy over the counter?
♦ Do you take any herbal remedies or supplements?
♦ Do you have any allergies to medications?
♦ Are you wearing any medication patches?
♦ Do you take any medicines that are prescribed by someone other than your GP, e.g. you obtain them through the hospital?
♦ Do you use any medicines such as inhalers, sprays, creams or eye drops?

When documenting the medicines reconciliation, it is useful to consider that this information will be used by the whole healthcare team and to think about whether all the information is there that you would want if you were to see that patient in the future.

Medication Review

Medication review is another component of effective medicines optimisation as it provides the opportunity to look holistically at all the medicines the patient is taking in a structured way. A medication review is defined as a 'structured, critical examination of a person's medicines with the objective of reaching an agreement with the person about treatment, optimising the impact of their medicines, minimising the number of medication related problems and reducing waste' (NICE 2015). There is a NICE quality standard in which one of the quality statements is that local healthcare providers should have in place ways of identifying those patients who would benefit from such a review (NICE 2016, Quality statement 6).

This quality standard highlights that the process of medication review is of particular relevance for older people and people of any age with polypharmacy and long-term health problems (NICE 2016). District nurse prescribers undertaking medication review should take into account the patient's views and understanding of their own medicines in a person-centred approach, and any views, concerns or understanding of the family or the carer. There should be a focus on any risk factors for developing any adverse reactions, such as a change in medicine regime, altered blood chemistry or dietary changes. There should be consideration of the safety and effectiveness of how the patient is using their prescribed medication and if it is being used as prescribed and in line with the current evidence base or national guideline for this medicine. District nurse prescribers should also consider what monitoring and follow-up processes need to be initiated following the medication review to ensure safety and efficacy of use.

Turn to **Chapter 3** to review history-taking and consultation.

Think about:

♦ Do you know where you would refer a patient for a structured medication review if you highlighted there were problems with their medication and it was beyond your scope of practice to deal with this?

Medicines Adherence

The concept of how patients use prescribed medicine – i.e. if they actually take the medicine once the consultation has ended and they are left to their own devices – is not new. There have been several different iterations of terms that have been used to describe this. You have probably heard the terms compliance, concordance and adherence all used. As with all uses of language to describe something that is inherently complex and multifactorial, there are challenges with getting it right. Compliance, for example, is no longer favoured because the word itself implies that patients should submit and be compliant with a particular medication regimen. This reinforces a paternalistic approach to medicine where the patient is somehow at fault if they do not 'comply' with the prescriber's instructions. Commonly in practice, the term adherence is used as it implies a greater degree of autonomy on the part of the patient. In this section we will be using the term adherence to talk about how patients use their medicines.

> **Definition of adherence:**
>
> 'The extent to which the patient's action matches the agreed recommendations' (NICE 2009).

Imagine the scenario. You have spent a long time completing your training to become an independent prescriber and have learnt all about the drugs in your scope of practice. You prescribe a medication for one of your patients based on the most up-to-date clinical practice and in line with clinical guidelines to help them stop smoking. You know that this will reduce the patient's long-term morbidity and risk of mortality due to their diagnosis of COPD. The next time you are at your base or able to access the GP practice, you see from the records that they have not been ordering the medication. What feelings will you experience – frustration, annoyance or maybe resignation as you know from experience that patients often don't take their medicines as prescribed?

In fact, data quoted in documents produced by the WHO (2003), the RPS (2015) and NICE (2009) show that:

♦ Despite medicines being the most common form of intervention to manage and treat ill health in the UK, particularly long-term conditions, it is estimated that 30–50% of medicines used in the treatment of long-term conditions are not used as prescribed.
♦ Only 16% of patients who are prescribed a new medicine take it as prescribed, experience no problems and receive as much information as they need.
♦ Ten days after starting a medicine, almost a third of patients are already non-adherent.
♦ Of these, 55% don't realise they are not taking their medicines correctly, whilst 45% are intentionally non-adherent.

♦ Between one-third and half of all prescribed medicines for long-term conditions are not being taken as recommended.

From this we can see that if your patient doesn't take the medicines you prescribe in the way you intend, then you are certainly not alone. The questions, then, are what are the reasons for this and what can you do as a prescriber to support adherence?

Think about:

♦ What reasons have you come across in practice for patients being non-adherent?
♦ Can you break these down at all into categories?

Looking at the data from the RPS (2015), there is one statement that can give us some insight into a key differentiating factor in reasons for non-adherence: '55% don't realise they are not taking their medicines correctly, whilst 45% are intentionally non-adherent'. So very roughly half of patients don't even mean to be non-adherent. These patients will need a very different approach compared to the other half who are intentionally not taking their medicines. You will therefore often see adherence categorised as unintentional or intentional.

Unintentional non-adherence is when the patient would like to follow the prescribed regime but is unable to. This can be for all sorts of reasons, such as a lack of understanding, inability to source the treatment or memory loss.

Intentional non-adherence is when there is a deliberate decision not to follow the treatment for whatever reason, due to beliefs or preference.

Supporting Patients Who Are Non-adherent

Case Study 11.1

You have an appointment with Mr Moses who is housebound due to poor health. When you start talking to him, you suspect that there is a problem with his adherence to his medication.

♦ How do you think you will be able to identify either intentional or unintentional non-adherence?
♦ What different ways are there for you to support a patient who is non-adherent?

Identifying patients who are unintentionally non-adherent:

It can be a challenge identifying these patients, as they believe they are adherent. They may be ordering their medicines and taking them, but they may not be taking them in the way that they are prescribed. This can lead to a loss of efficacy, an increase in side effects or problems with patient safety.

Change how you ask questions: Rephrasing questions can help. Some examples are given below.

Rather than asking 'Are you taking your medicines?', ask other questions such as 'How do you take your medicines?' or 'When do you take your medicines?'. For example, if a patient is taking simvastatin, it must be taken at night to produce an effect due to its pharmacological properties. In practice, patients can be unaware of this and they take it in the morning. So, they are taking the medicine, but it won't reduce their cholesterol and just puts them at risk of side effects.

Addressing the problem of patients forgetting: A common problem can be that patients intend to take their medicines but forget. Often patients don't want to disclose this information as they are embarrassed or feel that they are at fault. The questions you ask can help patients report non-adherence. Using open, non-judgemental questions can help patients be honest.

♦ Instead of asking 'Do you take all of your medicines all the time?', you could say 'Tell me about whether you have any problems remembering to take your medicines'.
♦ You can also ask in a way that does not apportion blame, by generalising, e.g. 'Lots of people I see have trouble remembering'.
♦ Explain why you are asking about this: 'If you forget to take your blood pressure medicine then you won't be getting the benefit, but we can look at maybe changing things to support you in reducing your blood pressure.'
♦ Asking about a specific timeframe can also help: 'Have you missed any of your medicines in the last week/month?' You can then go on to explore the reasons for this.

Looking at patients' medicines/ordering patterns: You may identify patients who are unintentionally non-adherent by looking at their medicines or ordering patterns. For example, if the patient is using a dossette box or blister pack, there may be missed days. If the patient is forgetting to order medicines, you may pick this up from their ordering patterns.

Checking whether patients can use their medicines: When medicines are administered via some kind of device, such as an inhaler, an eye drop or injection, patients can struggle to be adherent. Metered dose inhalers (MDIs) are notoriously difficult to use effectively. The coordination of breath and actuation is complex and this is why all patients should have their inhaler technique checked regularly. Through checking inhaler technique, unintentional non-adherence can be identified. Although well recognised for inhalers, regular review can also support patients using other devices.

Identifying patients who are intentionally non-adherent:

The first step in identifying intentional non-adherence is having a patient-centred approach to prescribing. This means encouraging patients to be able to discuss treatment options in a way that encourages the idea of informed adherence. The decision to be non-adherent may be influenced by many factors, such as beliefs around medicines in general, anxiety about a particular medication or a perception that the medication is not needed. It is only by encouraging the patient to talk about any factors that might influence their decision that you can support them in making an informed decision about adherence.

This means having an open approach that allows a frank discussion with patients about any concerns or doubts they may have. It also means discussing with patients their beliefs and perceptions about treatment and any specific barriers to adherence. Remember this is not a one-off conversation when treatment is initiated, as perceptions can change over time. Using open questions and a 'no-blame' approach is crucial when having these conversations.

Ideas for supporting patients who are unintentionally non-adherent:

♦ Consider changing the frequency of the medicine, e.g. switch from a three-times-daily to a once-daily regimen.

♦ Consider whether the timing is a problem, e.g. the patient takes all but one of their medicines in the morning or forgets to take their night-time medicine. Does the medicine have to be taken at night? If it does, can it be swapped for another medicine that can be taken in the morning (e.g. simvastatin must be taken at night, but atorvastatin can be taken at any time)?

♦ Do they need some help to remember, e.g. dossette boxes or even, if the situation warrants it, carers? There are also a whole range of apps that can be used that prompt patients to take medicines. These can be great for patients who have access to and are able to use smart phones.

♦ Would a change in the formulation or device used to administer the medicine help? For example, could the patient be adherent if they used a spacer or a breath-actuated inhaler?

♦ Provide sufficient information to the patient. This may need to be adapted to the needs of the patient, e.g. if the patient is blind, has a learning disability or English is their second language.

Ideas for supporting patients who are intentionally non-adherent:

♦ Discuss with the patient the underlying ideas, beliefs and values that have informed their decision not to take a medication.
♦ Address any factual inaccuracies that may be influencing this decision. For example, they may say they don't want to take a medicine because of a side effect that is not related to this medicine, e.g. evidence has shown the link between autism and vaccines to be untrue.
♦ Discuss whether other pharmacological or non-pharmacological options may align with the patient's views better, depending on the nature of the condition being treated.
♦ If side effects are causing the decision, then consider how to minimise these and balance the decision against the long-term benefit of the drug. This may include considering dose adjustments, managing the side effects or switching to another medicine that has a different side-effect profile.

The case study above illustrates some of the ways in which non-adherence can be identified and some ideas for support that can be provided to patients to support adherence. The challenge comes in that patients are all individual and the diversity of reasons for non-adherence is endless. There is also a lack of evidence about which interventions can increase adherence (NICE 2015), and so interventions should be tailored specifically to the patient. It is important to appreciate that if a patient makes a choice not to take a medicine, that is their right. Patients who have capacity have the right to make what we may consider to be unwise decisions. As a prescriber, your role is to make sure that this choice is based on all the evidence available about the risks and benefits. If you identify non-adherence and after a full discussion about the medication the patient decides they still do not want to take it, you must ensure that this conversation is fully documented. There should also be the option for the patient to revisit this decision, as values, beliefs and also perceptions of the risks and benefit can change over time.

The Challenge of Polypharmacy

NICE (2015) identifies that the average number of prescription items for any person in England was 19 per year in 2013, an increase from 13 items per person in 2003. The use of multiple medicines in an individual patient is referred to as 'polypharmacy'. With an increase in long-term conditions and multi-morbidity, coupled with an increasingly ageing population, this has become a key issue in prescribing practice for all prescribers.

Because of the increased risk of problems associated with the use of multiple medicines, the term polypharmacy has mainly been associated with negative connotations. Duerden et al. (2013) identified that polypharmacy is something that should be avoided in prescribing and healthcare practice where possible. It is, however, acknowledged that the challenge of prescribing in complex patients means that sometimes polypharmacy is appropriate, whilst at other times it is not. This has given rise to the terms appropriate polypharmacy and problematic polypharmacy.

Appropriate polypharmacy: Prescribing for an individual for complex or multiple conditions in circumstances where medicines use has been optimised and where the medicines are prescribed according to the best evidence (Duerden et al. 2013).

Problematic polypharmacy: The prescribing of multiple medicines inappropriately or where the intended benefits of the medicines are not realised (Duerden et al. 2013). This can include issues such as:

♦ Interactions with other medications
♦ Taking too many tablets, which the patient finds unacceptable (pill burden)
♦ Taking so many medicines that the patient cannot maintain the prescribed regime
♦ Medicines being prescribed to treat side effects of other medicines (the prescribing cascade)
♦ Not stopping medicines that are no longer needed.

Undertaking medication review in patients on multiple medicines can help to identify when polypharmacy is appropriate and when it is problematic. In some areas, GP practices may have pharmacists who can conduct in-depth reviews for patients on multiple medicines. Find out what services are available in the area where you work.

Turn to **Chapter 5** for more on prescribing in patients with co-morbidities.

Prescribing in Long-term Conditions

A long-term condition is defined as a condition that cannot be cured and is controlled by medicines and/or other treatments and therapies (Snodden 2010). The prevalence of long-term conditions in the UK has increased, and they are now the most common cause of death and disability in England (NICE 2015).

In 2015, within the UK, 17.5 million people were estimated to have a long-term condition and the number with multiple long-term conditions was estimated at 2.9 million people (NICE 2018). It makes sense that if a patient has one or more long-term conditions then they can be at risk of some the problems already discussed in this chapter, such as polypharmacy, non-adherence or errors if medicines reconciliation is not done on transfer of care.

Considerations for Optimising Medicines in Long-term Conditions:

♦ Ensure appropriate reviews take place to ensure medicines are still needed and address any problems with polypharmacy (see below)
♦ Check that medicines are still effective, e.g. analgesics are still providing adequate pain relief
♦ Check adherence
♦ Check that medicines are still appropriate as per guidance, as this can obviously change with time
♦ Ensure that any routine monitoring has been conducted
♦ Ensure that any new medicines prescribed for either an acute or chronic condition are compatible with existing management of the long-term condition
♦ Ensure medicines reconciliation has taken place at an appropriate time.

De-prescribing

So far we have talked about how we optimise medicines when they should be used. In this section we will talk in more detail about optimising medicines by stopping them. In recent years the term de-prescribing has come into common use in healthcare. This is an activity whereby medicines that are not appropriate for the patient are withdrawn in a safe way. This may be particularly useful in patients where there are increased risks, perhaps due to polypharmacy. However, all patients should have medicines de-prescribed that are not appropriate for them.

In practice it can be challenging to feel confident to stop medicines, due to lack of support on whether it is safe and effective to do this. There are some tools available that can help identify patients who may be on medicines inappropriately, for example the STOPP/START tool or the BEERs criteria. Alternatively, a medication review prompted by a range of situations could identify medicines that could be de-prescribed – e.g. medicines being ineffective or causing an ADR, or a change in treatment priorities (Jansen et al. 2016).

Toolkits to Support De-prescribing

As well as formularies and guidelines, there are toolkits available to assist prescribers in optimising medicines. These can assist in making safe decisions in managing high-risk medicines in medication reviews.

The STOPP/START toolkit (Cumbria Clinical Commissioning Group 2016) is designed to optimise prescribing specifically in older patients (65 years and over). This group is particularly at risk because of some of the physiological and pharmacological changes described in **Chapter 5**. This can make them more likely to be prescribed multiple medicines and to be at risk of ADRs and drug interactions. As with any patient prescribed multiple medicines, there can problems with adherence, either intentionally or unintentionally. The toolkit is designed to look at drugs prescribed in different body systems (e.g. cardiovascular, urinary), and as such is grouped in the same way that BNF chapters are. The risk/benefit of stopping or starting treatments is considered, along with key prescribing information (such issues around renal impairment). Whilst it is unlikely you would be involved in completing a full medication review based on this tool, it is another source of support to inform your prescribing decisions.

Another similar screening tool focusing on reducing potentially inappropriate medicines (PIMs) prescribing in older patients is the BEERs criteria, also known as the BEERs list (American Geriatrics Society 2019). This includes lists of drugs broken down into the following five categories:

♦ Drugs that should be avoided by most older people (outside of hospice and palliative care settings)
♦ Drugs that should be avoided by older people with specific health conditions
♦ Drugs that should be avoided in combination with other treatments because of the risk for harmful 'drug-drug' interactions
♦ Drugs that should be used with caution because of the potential for harmful side effects
♦ Drugs that should be dosed differently for, or avoided altogether by, people with reduced kidney function, which impacts how the body processes medicine

One limitation with this is that it was developed by the American Geriatrics Society (AGS), so some of the medications included are not the same as those used in the UK.

Any decision to stop a medication should be based on the patient's physical functioning, co-morbidities, lifestyle and preferences (CQC 2018). It is crucial that this decision is made in collaboration with the patient, using a shared decision-making (SDM) approach (for more on this, see the SDM section later on in this chapter).

Ensuring Medicines Use is as Safe as Possible

In 2017, the WHO launched its third global patient safety challenge, 'medication without harm' (WHO 2017). The aim of this is to reduce harm from the 'global burden of severe and avoidable medication-related harm by 50% over five years' (WHO 2017). In response to this, research was commissioned in the UK that showed (NHS Improvement 2017):

♦ There are an estimated 237 million 'medication errors' per year in the NHS in England, with 66 million of these potentially clinically significant
♦ 'Definitely avoidable' adverse drug reactions collectively cost £98.5 million annually, contribute to approximately 1,700 deaths and are directly responsible for approximately 700 deaths per year

This shows that there is work to be done in improving medicines safety, another key principle of medicines optimisation (RPS 2013).

You will need to ensure you are aware of any policies and procedures in place to improve patient safety. Preventable adverse outcomes can be caused by errors which occur through a lack of knowledge, poor systems and protocols, competency deficits, poor communication and interruptions to the prescribing process. Robust professional and organisational systems can prevent errors in prescribing practice and minimise the risk of adverse outcomes.

Think about:

♦ How are prescribers in your area made aware of patient safety alerts issued by the NHS central alerting system (CAS)?
♦ Do you know what the National Reporting and Learning System (NRLS) is and how the information gathered from it is used locally? If you don't, go to: https://improvement.nhs.uk/resources/learning-from-patient-safety-incidents.
♦ How you will report and learn from patient safety incidents as a prescriber?

Turn to **Chapter 5** for information on identifying, managing and reporting ADRs via the Medicines Health and Regulatory Agency (MHRA) Yellow Card Scheme.

Shared Decision-Making (SDM)

Sharing decisions with patients about their care is not a new concept. How much this happened in practice was in the past to a large extent dependent on individual practitioners. National policy is changing this and pushing for SDM to be integrated into routine practice through the introduction of various legislative and contractual mechanisms. These include the NHS Health and Social Care Act 2012 and the NHS Constitution.

It also forms a key part of the NHS England's plans around making care personalised to the needs of the patient. **Figure 11.2** shows that SDM underpins care across the whole population in NHS England's comprehensive model of personalised care.

So, why is there such a focus on SDM?

Some of the reasons given by the King's Fund (Coulter and Collins 2011) are:

♦ Patients who are actively involved in decisions engage more in their treatment
♦ Patients want to be more involved
♦ This approach can reduce variations in clinical practice
♦ It underpins the philosophy of patient-centred care.

One of the problems with adopting this approach nationally is that there is confusion about what SDM actually is.

Definition: Shared Decision Making

The NHS England (2018) website defines SDM as:

'A collaborative process through which a clinician supports a patient to reach a decision about their treatment

The conversation brings together:

♦ The clinician's expertise, such as treatment options, evidence, risks and benefits
♦ What the patient knows best: their preferences, personal circumstances, goals, values and beliefs'.

This approach recognises the value of both parties in the consultation, with the patient's lived experience having a valid role to play in the decision-making process. This is combined with the expertise of the clinician to allow a decision to be reached.

The King's Fund identifies this as relying on three key components (Coulter and Collins 2011):

♦ Provision of reliable, balanced, evidence-based information outlining treatment, care or support options, outcomes and uncertainties
♦ Decision support counselling with a clinician or health coach to clarify options and preferences
♦ A system for recording, communicating and implementing the patient's preferences.

Think about:

♦ How might you integrate SDM into your practice?

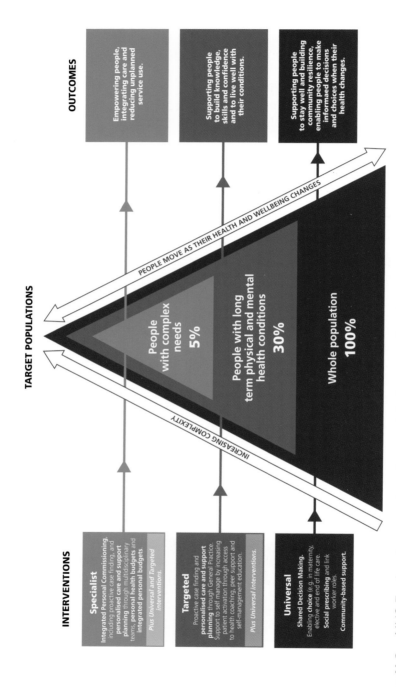

Figure 11.2 – NHS England comprehensive model of personalised care: All age, whole population approach to personalised care

Source: NHS England (2018).

One challenge that prescribers find with this approach is how to discuss options with patients in the context of the evidence. If, for example, a patient needs an anti-hypertensive, how do you present the options and discuss what the risks and benefits are?

It can help to use a patient decision aid (PDA). These vary in format and may be written, accessed online or in DVD format. Some may have a greater depth of information than others. They should, however, have certain key information included in them, which is summarised in **Box 11.2**. From this, you can see that the PDA is more than just an information leaflet; it also should support the patient in identifying what is most important for them.

Because of the variability in the standard of PDAs being produced, the International Patient Decision Aid Standards (IPDAS) Collaboration was set up. This has produced a comprehensive checklist of standards that PDAs should conform to.

To view the full checklist, go to the IPDAS website: http://ipdas.ohri.ca.

Think about:

♦ Do you know if there are any PDAs used by your practice currently?
♦ If you don't know, who could you ask to find this out?
♦ Think of any areas in your scope of practice where using PDAs might support SDM.

Box 11.2 – Summary of key questions that should be used to evaluate a PDA

♦ Does it include a list of the options available to the patient (remember that doing nothing should be one of the options)?
♦ Are the outcomes of each of the options discussed, including discussion of probabilities of positive or negative outcomes?
♦ Does it include ways to support clarification of patient's values?
♦ When was the resource produced (so you can assess whether the information is still up to date)?
♦ Who was involved in producing the PDA and what evidence was used (PDAs are produced internationally, so you need to ensure that the options link to UK guidance)?
♦ Is the PDA written in language that the patient will be able to read and understand?

One barrier to SDM identified by clinicians is patients not being prepared to engage with the process. You may have come across the type of statements outlined below:

> Prescriber: So, I've given you the treatment options, what medication do you think you should take?
> Patient: You're the expert. What do you think I should take?

Changing the style of consultation is a cultural shift not just for the prescriber but also for the patient. It is therefore important to think about how to prepare and engage patients with this approach. The Making Good Decisions in Collaboration (MAGIC) programme looked at how SDM could be made part of routine practice in a range of care settings. The evaluation report (King et al. 2013) looked at a whole range of facilitators and barriers to making this happen. One factor it identified was that in order for patients to be able to participate in this process, they need support.

The NHS has produced a patient information leaflet adapted from the MAGIC evaluation. It explains how and why patients would benefit from becoming involved in decisions about their care. It encourages patients to Ask 3 Questions to help them make choices about their treatment. Access this leaflet and see how you can you use it to help patients be involved in decision making. It is available at: https://www.pat.nhs.uk/downloads/patient-information-leaflets/other/Ask%203%20Questions%20Leaflet.pdf. Various NHS organisations also have their own versions of leaflets based on Ask 3 Questions. Find out if your local area has one.

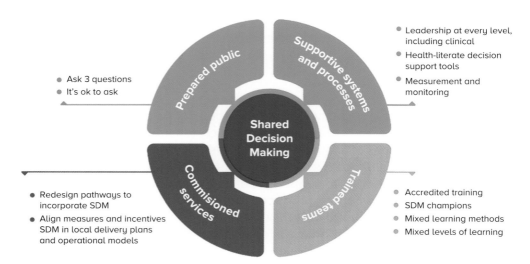

Figure 11.3 – NHS England: What good shared decision making looks like – for the system

Source: NHS England (2018).

Figure 11.3 summarises what NHS England sees SDM looking like as a system-wide approach, with four key domains:

1. Prepared public
2. Supportive systems and processes
3. Appropriately commissioned services
4. Appropriately trained teams

Think about:

Based on the NHS England domains in **Figure 11.3**, how are you going to:

♦ Prepare your patients for SDM?
♦ Use health-literate decision support tools?
♦ Find out whether any locally commissioned services integrate SDM already?
♦ Find out whether there is any local training available so you can develop your knowledge and skills?

Motivational Interviewing

Throughout this chapter there has been a focus on the patient, since how they engage with using medicines is a key factor in optimising therapeutic outcomes. When prescribing, it is important to remember that often you will be having conversations with patients that mean they will have to make a change in their behaviour.

This may be changing their daily routine to accommodate adherence to a medication. For example, if a diuretic like furosemide is prescribed, the patient will need to stay near to toilet facilities because of the diuresis. This may mean missing a social event they usually attend. It can also be linked to profound life changes, like losing weight or stopping smoking.

Motivational interviewing is a style of consulting that aims to support patients in changing their behaviour. It was born out of the recognition that simply telling patients they needed to change did not work. The initial group of patients that it was developed in during the 1980s was patients with severe substance misuse problems. Medicines can play a role in supporting these patients, as there are a multitude of social and behavioural factors that are key for patients to overcome their addictions. Since then, its use has expanded to a whole range of other clinical areas, such as for patients with heart failure, COPD and diabetes.

The ethos behind motivational interviewing is to help the patient to identify and engage with their own intrinsic motivation to change. The role of the clinician is therefore guiding the patient to identify for themselves why they think they should change rather than fulfilling the more traditional didactic role of telling them why they should change. The clinician can then help patients define their goals and plan with them how they might achieve them.

This is broken down into four key processes:

Engaging: This is where a working therapeutic relationship is developed, which is an essential prerequisite for the other processes. This does not just involve being nice to the patient; it is about developing trust through finding out what is important to the patient through the use of open questions and reflective listening.

Focusing: This is where there is a focus on an agenda and identifying the goals the patient may wish to achieve.

Evoking: Once the change goals have been focused in on, the next process is to evoke the patient's motivation on why and how they might achieve this.

Planning: If the patient is ready to move beyond why they want to make change to the detail of how this might happen, then the discussion can be had about formulating a specific plan of action.

To develop the skills needed to be effective at this style of consulting, you will need to undertake further reading and ideally training. A good starting point is the article 'Motivational Interviewing: The competent novice' (Rollnick et al. 2010), which gives an overview of simple ways to integrate this into your practice. If you want more detail, then Rollnick and Miller (2013) provide a comprehensive guide with useful practice examples. There are also various online resources available that you may find useful – for example, the Royal College of Nursing (RCN) has resources available at: https://www.rcn.org.uk/clinical-topics/supporting-behaviour-change/motivational-interviewing. In some practices there may be prescribers who are already using this technique to support their patients, such as nurses providing smoking cessation services or GPs seeing routine patients. You may be able to observe their consultations to support your own development.

Case Study 11.2

Imagine you go to review Mrs O'Neill following discharge from hospital after an exacerbation of COPD. You haven't met her before. You see from her medical records that she is a smoker.

- ♦ How will you engage with this patient to build a therapeutic relationship?
- ♦ How will you focus on identifying the patient's agenda and her change goals around their smoking?
- ♦ How will you evoke her motivation for change?
- ♦ If the patient expresses a readiness for change, how will you support her in planning this?

Think about:

♦ What groups of patients do you work with where this approach may be of use?
♦ How are you going to develop your skills in this technique?

Conclusion

In this chapter, we have explored the process and concept of medicines optimisation from the prescribing perspective of district nurse practice. This is a big area that underpins a whole range of practice. It will take time and experience to gain confidence in all the ways of supporting your patients to get the best out of their medicines. However, having in mind the Royal Pharmaceutical Society's (2013) four guiding principles of medicines optimisation can help keep you focused on embedding patient-centred, evidence-based, safe and effective prescribing into your practice.

Key Points of This Chapter

♦ Medicines optimisation is essential to ensure effective use of medicines, particularly in the management of long-term conditions and multi-morbidity, due to a higher incidence of polypharmacy.
♦ Polypharmacy should be appropriate, and patients on multiple medicines should be monitored and reviewed regularly.
♦ Safety is paramount in prescribing practice and should be ensured at all times in medicines use, but in particular when patients are transferred from one care setting to another.
♦ Medicines optimisation should be patient-centred and any decisions should be made in partnership with patients using appropriate communication and decision support. This should help improve patient experience and outcomes, as well as safety.
♦ Decisions should always take an evidence-based approach.
♦ Working collaboratively with other healthcare practitioners and prescribers, with effective communication, can help support this process, as can the use of evidence-based toolkits to support prescribing practice.

References and Further Reading

American Geriatrics Society (2019) Beers Criteria® update expert panel. American Geriatrics Society 2019 updated AGS Beers Criteria® for potentially inappropriate medication use in older adults. *Journal of the American Geriatrics Society* 67(4): 674–694.

British National Formulary (BNF) (2017) *The British National Formulary 74, September 2017–March 2018*. London: The BMJ Group.

Coulter, A. and Collins, A. (2011) *Making Shared Decision Making a Reality: No Decision About Me Without Me*. London: The King's Fund.

Cumbria Clinical Commissioning Group (2016) The STOPP/START toolkit; supporting medication review. Available at: https://www.herefordshireccg.nhs.uk/your-services/medicines-optimisation/prescribing-guidelines/deprescribing/748-stopp-start-herefordshire-october-2016/file (accessed 26 February 2020).

Department of Health and Social Care (2016*) The Report of the Short Life Working Group on Reducing Medication-Related Harm*. Available at: https://assets.publishing.service.gov.uk/government/uploads/system/uploads/attachment_data/file/683430/short-life-working-group-report-on-medication-errors.pdf.

Deveugele, M., Derese, A., De Maesschalck, S. et al. (2005) Teaching communication skills to medical students, a challenge in the curriculum? *Patient Education and Counselling* 58(3): 265–270.

Duerden, M., Avery, T. and Payne, R. (2013) *Polypharmacy and Medicines Optimisation: Making it Safe and Sound*. London: The King's Fund.

Elliott, R. A., Camacho, E., Campbell, F. et al. (2018) Prevalence and economic burden of medication errors in the NHS in England. Policy Research Unit in Economic Evaluation of Health & Care Interventions (EEPRU). Available at: http://www.eepru.org.uk/wp-content/uploads/2018/02/eepru-report-medication-error-feb-2018.pdf.

Jansen, J., Naganathan, V., Carter, S. M. et al. (2016) Too much medicine in older people? Deprescribing through shared decision making. *British Medical Journal* 353–2893.

King, E., Taylor, J., Williams, R. et al. (2013) The MAGIC programme: Evaluation: An independent evaluation of the MAGIC (Making good decisions in collaboration) improvement programme. London: Health Foundation.

Matthys, J., Elwyn, G., van Nuland, M. et al. (2009) Patients' ideas, concerns, and expectations (ICE) in general practice: Impact on prescribing. *British Journal of General Practice* 59(558): 29–36.

Miller, W.R. and Rollnick, S. (2008) *Motivational Interviewing in Healthcare: Helping Patients Change Behaviour*. New York: Guilford Press.

National Institute for Health and Clinical Excellence (NICE) (2009) *Medicines Adherence: Involving Patients in Decisions about Prescribed Medicines and Supporting Adherence*. London: NICE.

National Institute for Health and Clinical Excellence (NICE) (2015) *Medicines Optimisation: The Safe and Effective Use of Medicines to Enable the Best Possible Outcomes*. London: NICE.

National Institute for Health and Clinical Excellence (NICE) (2016) *Medicines Optimisation QS120*. London: NICE.

National Institute for Health and Clinical Excellence (NICE) (2018) Medicines optimisation, quality standard. Available at: https://www.nice.org.uk/guidance/qs120/resources/medicines-optimisation-pdf-75545351857861.

National Institute for Health and Clinical Excellence (NICE) (2019) Key therapeutic topic [KTT23] shared decision making. Available at: https://www.nice.org.uk/advice/ktt23

National Patient Safety Agency (NPSA) (2010) *National Reporting and Learning System*. London: National Patient Safety Agency.

Neighbour, R. (1987) *The Inner Consultation: How to Develop Effective and Intuitive Consulting Style.* Lancaster: MTP Press.

NHS England (2018) Shared decision making summary guide. Available at: https://www.england.nhs.uk/wp-content/uploads/2019/01/shared-decision-making-summary-guide-v1.pdf.

NHS England and MHRA (2014) *Patient Safety Alert: Stage Three Directive, Improving Medication Error Incident Reporting and Learning.* London: NHS England.

NHS Improvement (2014) Learning from patient safety incidents. Available at: https://improvement.nhs.uk/resources/learning-from-patient-safety-incidents.

NHS Improvement (2017) National medicines safety programme. Available at: https://improvement.nhs.uk/resources/national-medicines-safety-programme.

Nunes, V., Neilson, J., O'Flynn, N. et al. (2009) *Clinical Guidelines and Evidence Review for Medicines Adherence: Involving Patients in Decisions about Prescribed Medicines and Supporting Adherence.* London: National Collaborating Centre for Primary Care and Royal College of General Practitioners.

Pendleton, D. (1984) *The Consultation – An Approach to Learning and Teaching.* Oxford: Oxford University Press.

Pendleton, D. (2003) *The New Consultation: Developing Doctor-Patient Communication.* Oxford: Oxford University Press.

Royal Pharmaceutical Society (RPS) (2013) *Medicines Optimisation: Helping Patients Make the Most of Their Medicines.* London: RPS.

Silverman, J., Kurtz, S. and Draper, J. (2013) *Skills for Communicating with Patients.* Boca Raton: CRC Press.

Snodden, J. (2010) *Case Management for Long-Term Conditions: Principles and Practice for Nurses.* Chichester: Blackwell Publishing.

Specialist Pharmacy Service (SPS) (2015) A patient centred approach to polypharmacy. NHS. Available at: https://www.sps.nhs.uk/wp-content/uploads/2014/12/Patient20Centred20Approach20to20Polypharmacy20summary20formerly20seven20steps.pdf.

Specialist Pharmacy Service (SPS) (2017) Improving the quality of medicines reconciliation. A best practice resource and toolkit. NHS. Available at: https://www.sps.nhs.uk/wp-content/uploads/2015/06/Medicines_Reconciliation_Best_Practice_Standards_Toolkit_Vs1.1_June-15-links-updated-Aug-17.pdf.

UK Medicines Information (UKMi) North West (2015) *NICE Bites: Medicines Optimisation (NG5).* No. 74. Liverpool: UKMi.

World Health Organization (WHO) (2003) *The World Health Report 2003: Shaping the Future.* Geneva: World Health Organization.

World Health Organization (WHO) (2017) Patient safety: The third WHO Global Patient Safety Challenge: Medication without harm. Available at: https://www.who.int/patientsafety/medication-safety/en.

Chapter 12
Reflective Practice: An Introduction or Refresher

Amanda Blaber and Hannah Ingram

In This Chapter

- Introduction
- Defining 'professional practice'
- Sources of expectation as a professional
- What constitutes 'advanced practice' for the district nurse?
- What is the purpose of reflection on your prescribing practice?
- Why write up reflections on prescribing?
- Commonly cited barriers to written reflection
- Ideas on how to make your reflections meaningful
- Reflective models
- Reflexivity versus reflection
- Clinical supervision or person-centred development?
- Conclusion
- Key points of this chapter
- References and further reading
- Useful websites.

Introduction

This chapter sets the context of professionalism in relation to advanced practice and your role as a district nurse independent prescriber. It will concentrate on ways to commence reflection and integrate this into your everyday practice. For many of you, reflection will already be a part of your everyday practice; for others it may be less formal or effective.

As people, we reflect for a large majority of our day, usually without consciously recognising that we are doing so. As professionals, we reflect at the time of care giving or 'in action', as Schön suggests (1983), whilst deciding on our interpersonal approach and communication, assessment and treatment. Our reflections affect our decision-making process and patient outcome. Much of this occurs automatically without us pausing and saying to ourselves 'now let me reflect'. We certainly think about people we have cared for after the event – 'reflection on action', as Schön (1983) suggests.

For many of you, this chapter will provide a refresher of the key concepts of reflective practice; for others it may present alternative options and new approaches to consider. One chapter cannot provide the depth and detail provided by specific textbooks on the subject of reflection, so should be considered as an introduction to the subject. Reflection will be explored as an individual process, moving on to more group-centred activities. A brief overview of some reflective models will also be provided. A specific prescribing reflective framework will be explained.

Reflection on practice is a key aspect of advancing practice and is an essential part of your continuing professional development (CPD). The inextricable nature of these two subjects is clear.

Defining 'Professional Practice'

'Professionalism' is a word commonly used in respect of all healthcare professions. The attributes of a profession and process of professionalisation have been the subject of much debate by sociologists and psychologists and have evolved over time. It is generally agreed that in order to be a 'legitimate' profession, there are several commonly agreed characteristics for any occupation to aspire to:

♦ To have their own specialised body of knowledge and related theories, gained through a higher education route
♦ Having control, autonomy and accountability to define boundaries and the nature of work
♦ Having a code of ethics which regulates relationships between professions and professionals and their clients
♦ Having a monopoly on their area of practice, i.e. no other health professional is able to perform the role.

The ongoing process of 'professionalisation' of the nursing profession reflects the points made above. Professionalism is an interesting debate, which probably raises more questions than can be answered. For example:

♦ Are roles within healthcare, like that that of an advanced practitioner, developing in complexity/diversity to satisfy societal demands of what the public expect healthcare professionals to be able to do?
♦ Are district nursing roles being extended and developed so that they can be utilised to 'plug the gap' of not enough doctors?
♦ Are allied healthcare professionals who are not doctors being used as a source of cheaper labour?
♦ Are advanced roles being developed to progress the professionalisation of the district nursing profession?

The questions are innumerable, with interesting social and professional debates to be had. The debate is worth initiating to ensure the district nursing profession is clear about future progress and developments.

Certainly, district nurses employed in advanced roles and those outside traditional areas of employment are at the forefront of challenging role boundaries and are continuing to define 'professional practice'.

Sources of Expectation as a Professional

Using the term 'professional' comes with certain expectations of you as a registered healthcare professional (Jasper and Rosser 2013). There are numerous sources of these expectations; see **Box 12.1**.

As a registrant and advanced practitioner, you should know the characteristics of a profession, and should meet the expectations that are incumbent upon you as a registered district nurse. This includes demonstrating the knowledge, skills and behaviours expected of you in your professional role. As an independent prescriber, you should ensure that you are fully cognisant of your professional practice responsibilities, which is why this chapter has briefly reviewed what

---

Box 12.1 – Sources of professional expectation

1. The government – via social, health and economic policy which determines a district nurse's role
2. The legal system – as the profession is regulated by law, district nurses are required to act lawfully, both personally and professionally
3. Employers – who decide organisational roles
4. Service users – who have expectations and first-hand experience of how district nurses act and execute their duties
5. The general public and medics – who are responsible for constructing an image of the profession
6. Colleagues – who set the culture by their own practice and actions, becoming role models for those entering the profession.
7. Other professions – who have their own views on the roles and functions of district nurses
8. Registering and professional body – the Nursing and Midwifery Council (NMC), which works on behalf of its members to move the profession forward and also provides many publications that registrants are required to understand and abide by. Examples of a few district nurse-specific documents are: Maybin et al. (2016); NMC (2001); Queen's Nursing Institute (2015).

'professional practice' means. The parameters described in Box 12.1 provide guidance for a practitioner's professional development. Points 1–8 in Box 12.1 may act as a starting point for analysing practice, identifying good practice and assessing your own development needs.

Any profession's standards and codes are broad in nature and attempt to encompass all given situations that the professional may find themselves in. It can be argued that standards and codes may be quite restrictive for a professional working within an advanced scope of practice. There is potential for professional inertia. Staff working in the NHS are familiar with the 6 Cs, with courage and compassion urged to be at the forefront of our practice and decision making, yet on occasions this is juxtaposed with restrictive professional standards. It is clear that the professional bodies are acting in the best interests of the public and professionals they represent. However, the more 'advanced' the professional becomes, the more professional opinion, knowledge, experience, expertise and a whole host of other aspects are part of their everyday decision making. Professionalism is about working within your professional scope, whilst also being brave enough to select the best option for your patient and society.

A particularly pertinent aspect of advanced district nurse practice is the professional decision *not* to do something in any given situation. Advanced practitioners and independent prescribers use their knowledge, experience and expertise in all situations to make the best decision for their patient. In some cases, this will not involve skills application or prescribing. As some of the previous chapters have highlighted, knowing when not to prescribe is equally, if not more, important than the action of prescribing.

Before discussing several ways to do this, it is worth exploring the concept of advanced practice from a district nurse perspective.

 Turn to **Chapter 3** for more on clinical decision making

What Constitutes 'Advanced Practice' for the District Nurse?

On a national basis in the UK, advanced practice is acknowledged as that which requires the practitioner to have completed a relevant master's degree. Studying at master's degree level (or level 7) challenges the individual to explore their practice area and associated subject complexities, and is a fundamental requirement of a professional moving towards working clinically in an advanced practice role. Advanced clinical practice is characterised by a high degree of autonomy and complex decision making, and encompasses the four pillars – clinical practice; leadership and management; research and development; and education – along with the demonstration of core capabilities and area-specific clinical competence. District nurses applying for a prescribing course may not hold a master's qualification, or be working towards one; they should, however, be working at an advanced level within the specialism of district nursing, where prescribing is central to the role to facilitate safe and effective timely patient-centred care.

With this level of academic standing comes self-awareness, supporting colleagues and advancing the profession. There are more aspects to advanced practice, but in order to be an effective advanced practitioner, many people find the process of reflection essential. The next section will propose some potential useful self-help ways to commence or continue your reflective abilities.

What is the Purpose of Reflection on Your Prescribing Practice?

Professional practice is full of dilemmas. The practitioner negotiates their way through these dilemmas on a daily basis; some are simpler than others. Schön describes the situation perfectly:

> 'In the varied topography of professional practice, there is a high, hard ground overlooking a swamp. On the high ground, manageable problems lend themselves to solutions through the use of researchbased theory and technique. In the swampy lowlands, problems are messy and confusing and incapable of technical solution. The irony of this situation is that the problems of the high ground tend to be relatively unimportant to individuals or society at large, however great their technical interest may be, while in the swamp lie the problems of greatest human concern. The practitioner is confronted with a choice. Shall he remain on the high ground where he can solve relatively unimportant problems according to his standards of rigor, or shall he descend to the swamp of important problems where he cannot be rigorous in any way he knows how to describe'.

(Schön 1987, p. 1)

In some ways, this refers back to the earlier discussion about the expectations of a professional and professional body regulation. The question is what can professionals do about the 'swampy lowlands'? An aspiring advanced district nurse should be intrigued by, engaged with and courageous enough to delve into the swampy lowlands. In these difficult situations, reflection is fundamental and is an essential part of the process to tease out the complexities, explore the possibilities and discover the truth about themselves, their colleagues and the profession to which they belong.

Incidents/events 'bug' our heads, so writing may be a way for us to deal with them effectively, professionally and developmentally. In any new role,

> ## Think about:
>
> How often would you say your thoughts or reflections are meaningful?
>
> Does just thinking about something help you personally?
>
> Does reflecting upon something help you improve your care in the future?
>
> Has reflecting on an incident or patient encounter ever helped you improve an outcome for a patient or helped you focus on your own CPD?

professionals will naturally reflect more earlier on, until they feel they have worked through the novice stage (Benner 2000). Gradually becoming more confident and competent as learning progresses, the end point is that of expert in this specific role. As a prescriber, you need to seriously consider using a structured written approach to reflection as one means of improving your practice. Perhaps the first step, if you are new to reflection, is to get started; some ideas follow in this chapter.

As healthcare professionals, it is usual that we are troubled by negative thoughts, but written reflection should also be used for positive outcomes and as a means to sharing best practice. As you will be aware, reflection is a means to assist the decision-making process, and can improve patient safety and quality of care. It forms a large part of nurses' CPD requirements and can form a vital part of your own professional development if it is meaningful.

Why Write up Reflections on Prescribing?

As healthcare professionals, we recognise our responsibilities to keep records for ourselves and as part of our role in maintaining our patients' safety whilst they are in our care and beyond. However, we are often not good at writing about ourselves or our practice, which is equally important in our professional responsibility and development.

Writing a series of reflections as a newly qualified independent prescriber gives a permanence to your thoughts, feelings, practice and stage of development. This is more useful to you than transient thoughts, which are not recorded in any way. The passage of time means your thoughts are usually lost. What may eventually become a reflective experience may start as a series of practice or case notes whilst you are working – an example of reflection-in-action. It may be that you later wish, for your own personal development, to reflect more deeply on an aspect of your case notes, where a written reflection would be more suitable and become a more permanent and useful record.

Writing in a reflective way may end up becoming a mixture of formats, such as a reflective log (Jasper 2008) or a structured account using a model.

It depends on the purpose at hand as to which tool is most suitable. Your reflections may be nostalgic (for you to look back on years later), private or emotive, or may act as a form of communication to others, for example via debrief. Written reflections can contribute to decision making if you encounter a similar situation again.

Commonly Cited Barriers to Written Reflection

There is a culture in some healthcare professions where anything to do with practice should be undertaken in paid work time. It may be viewed that this culture is at odds with the concept of life-long learning. Despite the NMC advocating the importance of enough time in a registrant's working day to be able to reflect on their practice (Nursing Times News Desk 2019), the process of life-long learning is not the employer's responsibility, but the registrants'. There will always be little or no time available in a working day for busy healthcare professionals to reflect effectively. The key word here is 'effectively'. We can think things through at the time or after the event, but are our efforts effective and reflective enough for us to truly say we have learnt from the experience or patient encounter? The ability of an individual to address their own shortcomings and lack of knowledge or to learn from an experience depends on their own personal insight and self-awareness. We take advantage of learning opportunities as they come our way, across the course of a day, but there will be times when an individual wishes to spend more time afterwards exploring, learning and reflecting on a specific aspect.

Many professionals cite time as a barrier to reflecting. Some people may find it hard to accept that it may be worth spending some of their own time away from the working environment on meaningful reflection. To those people I would ask the following question: if something from your working day is bugging your head, how much of your own time have you given it anyway? Would it have been a more efficient use of your downtime to log, write a case study or write reflectively, which may have resolved your nagging doubts and questions? As already mentioned, means of reflection can take different forms, and individuals need to explore what works best for them and suits the situation that requires exploring.

Ideas on How to Make Your Reflections Meaningful

Many of us have been required to write a written reflection as an academic piece of work at one time or another, which forms part of the assessment process. Some people will have found this process quite cathartic, while others may have found it annoying and not at all useful. Writing for an assessment is very different from writing for your own personal reasons, whether they be emotive or developmental.

You need to be ready to write reflectively; only you can see its benefits. Some key points that theorists on reflection, such as Bolton (2005, 2010), Jasper (2008, 2013; Jasper et al. 2013) and Rolfe et al. (2001), deem to be vital are as follows:

♦ Commitment from you is required in order to get the most from the reflective process
♦ You need to make time for yourself
♦ It will work best if you are self-aware; this may require additional work (the NHS leadership academy website has some useful exercises)
♦ It cannot be undertaken quickly and results may not be immediate
♦ You need to be honest and open in your writing
♦ You must want to learn from your experiences. Initially, when you begin to write, you may find yourself out of your comfort zone. You may also have this sense when you commence your role of independent prescriber. When you write more reflectively, you may be able to recognise tangible results from yourself and from professional exploration. This should enhance your prescribing practice
♦ You may need to explore a subject in depth in order to achieve the level of understanding required of your new role as an independent prescriber and work towards becoming more confident and competent
♦ During your depth of exploration, you may also explore your relationships inside and outside of the work environment, wider societal issues and the culture of the health service and your profession. The reflective process should not be restrictive.

There will be times when you need to write reflections for academic or CPD purposes. It is not necessarily the purpose of this chapter to discuss reflection in relation to academic assessment. Many experts on reflective writing (Bolton and Delderfield 2018; Jasper et al. 2013) agree that there are various strategies for reflective writing. They agree that it can be described as a continuum, with analytical reflective writing at one end and creative writing at the other.

Analytical strategies are normally used when others are likely to see your writing. In such circumstances, models of reflection may be useful to come to an end action point. Other examples of analytical reflective writing strategies include:

♦ Critical incident analysis
♦ Using frameworks or models
♦ Strengths, weaknesses, opportunities and threats (SWOT) analysis
♦ Report writing
♦ Learning outcomes
♦ Journal writing/logs.

Towards the more creative end of the reflective writing continuum are:

♦ Writing to someone else
♦ Writing unseen letters or emails
♦ Storytelling/poetry.

As a general rule, the more creative the strategy used, the less analysis is achieved. Creative examples may be useful if you are trying to initiate discussion with others on a subject or to capture your own unique version of an event. Which strategy you choose will depend on the following:

♦ Why you want to write – assessment or personal
♦ Who is likely to see it – personal or public
♦ What happened – personal or professional development
♦ What you want to achieve from the reflective experience
♦ If there is anyone else involved
♦ If there are any professional/ethical issues.

Below are some of the short-term goals that may help you get started on reflective writing and with an outcome that is meaningful rather than functional.

Short-term Reflection Ideas to Get You Started

If you perceive time to be a barrier in reflecting, these ideas may help. Jasper and Mooney (2013) and Bolton and Delderfield (2018) believe that these techniques can be used on a daily basis and should not be seen as additional to your work. The point is to make a note of what happens during your day for potential reflective use at a later date. Below are two of their suggested techniques.

Three a Day (Jasper and Mooney 2013)

Think about and write down the three most important things that happened *to you* during a shift. If this becomes tedious, you can alter the focus, by considering what you enjoyed the most, what you enjoyed the least, what you learnt during the shift, what challenged you the most, things you did not know, things you felt confident about, things you felt inadequate while doing and things that did (or did not) go as planned. The list can keep growing – things that come into your head are the most important. Jotting them down during your shift may help when you reflect after it is over.

Time-limited Stimuli (Bolton and Delderfield 2018)

It may be hard at first. Set yourself a short period of time, say six minutes. Sit with a pen and paper, and write down whatever comes into your head. It appears that having to commit something to paper stimulates the brain to bring experiences to your mind from its depths. This can then form the basis of your reflection should you so wish.

Medium-term Reflection Goals

Keep a reflective log or journal that you commit to writing once a week, making a pact with yourself to do so.

Or set time aside each week to review what has happened and record your feelings and reflections.

Or identify one event per week that stands out in your mind to explore in depth each week. You must be prepared to delve deeper into the experience and challenge yourself to learn more and view it from others' perspectives.

Spend no longer than one hour per week on the above options. If you are consistent and apply yourself, over time, all of these small 'chunks' will provide you with the following:

♦ Identification of your learning needs as an independent prescriber.
♦ Learning from your experiences
♦ Developed action plans from your experiences
♦ The possibility of solving problems in practice that have been around a while.
♦ A greater understanding of the way you work as a professional
♦ An ongoing record of your development as an independent prescriber
♦ Material you can build on from a practice development perspective and which may form the basis of problem-based learning with other colleagues who are experiencing the new role of prescribing for themselves
♦ A professional portfolio, created in a gradual manner
♦ Evidence of achieving your CPD standard.

Reflection is a process that is as important to a professional as other activities, such as record-keeping or keeping up to date with developments in practice. It should be an integral part of who you are as an advanced paramedic and an independent prescriber.

Long-term Reflection Goals

If you reach the stage of long-term goals, you will probably be in the habit of reflecting and will find that it comes very naturally to you and is part of who you are. One simple way to continue your reflective writing is to review your previous writing. Over time and with your prescribing experience accumulating, reviewing your earlier reflections should be an interesting exercise, enabling you to clearly see your journey and your triumphs, and possibly allowing you to identify issues that were important back then and that may still be relevant. You may wish to use some of your writing to share with others or use it to stimulate discussion in a professional group situation. The writing that you wish to share will certainly form part of your professional portfolio.

Reflective Models

Remember, there are no rules in relation to reflection. It is yours. As mentioned earlier, reflective models are useful when you require a structure and format for a reflective exercise, usually as part of an assessment process. A model approach may be useful for CPD or a portfolio presentation. The following section will provide an overview of some commonly used models, with details of where to find more information in the reference list at the end of the chapter (see Table 12.1).

Some of the models in **Table 12.1** may be familiar. The table represents a small but varied selection of the numerous models that are available for you to use. The most important factor is that you take the time to research and find a model that suits you personally and suits the purpose for which you intend to use it.

Box 12.2 has used some of the sections/prompts that are advocated by the Council of Wales Deanery (2018) for GP prescribing CPD framework, and examples of the original framework can be found on its website (see the references section for details). However, the prescribing framework presented in **Box 12.2** has been developed to be more suited to the early career prescriber.

Box 12.2 provides a suggested means for district nurses to begin reviewing their prescribing practice. It is hoped that district nurses will reflect on the medications they have prescribed for their patients on a regular basis in order to develop their prescribing practice and expertise. This framework provides prompts for the prescriber to consider during their reflection, which is important in roles that are new to an individual. As the prescriber becomes more competent, they will become less reliant on the prompts and will be able to reflect in their own unique way, probably using a recognised model of reflection.

Think about:

Are there any other prompts/questions that you would add to the framework in **Box 12.2**?

Reflexivity versus Reflection

In the course of your studies, you may hear the term 'reflexivity' mentioned. Experts on reflection provide clear definitions of the two, which are worth making clear in this chapter. Bolton (2010, p. 13) defines reflection as 'learning and developing through examining what we think happened on any occasion, and how we think others perceived the event and us, opening our practice to scrutiny by others, and studying data and texts from the wider sphere'.

Bolton (2010) suggests that reflexivity is somewhat deeper in terms of the reflective process and is more of an internal examination of us as individuals. This is perhaps one of the more meaningful definitions of reflexivity: 'What are the mental, emotional and value structures which allowed me to lose attention and make that error?' (Bolton 2010, p. 14). This focus on the negative needs to be balanced with positive reflections and celebrations of good practice and positive experiences.

Bolton (2010) suggests that this deep questioning is omitted if the practitioner undertakes the reflective process as a problem-solving exercise of: what happened; why; what did I think and feel; and how can I do it better next time?

Table 12.1 – Examples of some models of reflection

Name	Year	Title	Key concepts
Gibbs	1988	Reflective cycle	Six cyclical steps ◆ Description – what happened? ◆ Feelings – what were you thinking and feeling? ◆ Evaluation – what was good and bad about the experience? ◆ Analysis – what else can you make of the situation? ◆ Conclusion – what else could you have done? ◆ Action plan – if it arose again, what would you do?
Kolb	1984	Experiential learning theory	Works on two levels: four-stage cycle of learning and four separate learning styles *Four-stage cycle of learning:* ◆ Concrete experience or 'Do' – learner actively experiences an activity in practice ◆ Observation and reflection or 'Observe' – reflective observation – learner consciously reflects back on the experience ◆ Forming abstract concepts or 'Thinks' – learner attempts to conceptualise a theory or model of what is observed ◆ Active experimentation or 'Plan' – learner tries to plan how to test a model or theory, or plan a forthcoming experience

		Four learning styles: ◆ Assimilators – learn better when presented with sound logical theories to consider ◆ Convergers – learn better when provided with practical application of concepts and theories ◆ Accommodators – learn better when provided with hands-on experience ◆ Divergers – learn better when allowed to observe and collect a wide range of information
Johns	1995	Model of reflection	Based on the work of Carper (1978) Five cue questions arranged cyclically: ◆ Description of the experience – describe it and identify the significant factors ◆ Reflection – what was I trying to achieve and what were the consequences? ◆ Influencing factors – what factors, such as external/internal/knowledge, affected my decision making? ◆ Could I have dealt with it better? What other choices did I have and what might have been their consequences?

(continued)

Table 12.1 – Examples of some models of reflection (continued)

Name	Year	Title	Key concepts
			Learning – what will change because of this experience and how did I feel? How has this experience changed my ways of knowing:
			◆ Empirics – scientific ◆ Ethics – moral knowledge ◆ Personal – self-awareness ◆ Aesthetics – the art of 'what we do', our own experiences
			Johns' (2017) textbook contains other useful healthcare-related ideas for reflective practice
Bolton	2010	'Through the mirror' reflective practice writing model	Developed on the basis that all our actions are founded on our personal ethical values. 'We are what we do, rather than what we say we are' (Bolton 2010, p. 4)
			Writing 'through the mirror' is intuitive and spontaneous, like producing a first draft of an essay. These writings can then form the basis of discussion for confidential trusted forums or can be used by ourselves to learn more about *who* and *what* we are in practice. It provides insight into why we act as we do. The process can be unsettling and uneasy. It has been compared to mindfulness
			It is never good enough to say 'I don't have time to do X' or 'I did that because my senior told me to'. In healthcare and in life in general, there is much that is out of our control. But we are all responsible for our own actions

			If the concepts of this model are embraced, it has the potential to help you explore and 'question everything, turning your world inside out, outside in and back to front' (Bolton 2010, p. 11), hence the title 'through the mirror'
Ramsey	2005	Narrative learning cycle	Writing a story or narrative can provide some people who find reflection difficult with a way to express an experience with more confidence. Writing a story enables the use of 'she' or 'he' instead of 'I'. Some people will feel 'safer' and find this approach less personally revealing Fiction can slowly reveal episodes or combine things that happened at different times into one 'chunk' of writing. Your writing will still be from a deep professional experience and by 'retelling' may enable you to tackle issues 'head on', convey varying and various viewpoints (other than just your own) and reduce anxiety about reflecting on a painful incident

Box 12.2 – Reflective framework for early career prescribers

Name of drug	
Mode of action	Route
Dose/duration	Specify dose and length of prescription
Pharmacology	How does this drug work? If a patient asks you how it works or what it does, can you explain it? Review your associated anatomy and physiology
Why did I choose this drug?	Review your reasons Explore alternatives
What was I trying to achieve for this patient?	Review the patient's presenting complaint Review patient-specific issues, such as any other medication they may have been taking Consider possible drug interactions
Social history/ considerations	Considerations which may have been affected or enhanced For example, prescribing diuretics to a person with limited mobility. It may be very difficult for them to get to the toilet as often as needed. Thus, this may result in them not being concordant with your prescription
Positives of your drug choice	
Negatives of your drug choice	
Learning points	Review what you have learnt from thinking about this patient encounter
Action plan	What do I need to know in order to prescribe more effectively next time? What do I need to learn? What can I read? Who can I talk to?

Bolton suggests a 'through the mirror' model to assist practitioners with this self-exploration (see Table 12.1).

There are times in district nursing practice when discussing issues in a group situation is useful. The term 'debrief' is one that all healthcare workers are familiar with. However, the usefulness and success of such sessions vary enormously and they may leave more unanswered questions and worries than they solve. Very often debriefs are organised quickly, in response to an incident and run by an individual who does not have facilitative expertise or experience. They may also be part of a tick-box exercise, on behalf of the organisation, to say that a debrief was conducted. Often in district nursing practice, a debrief will happen on return to the office and can be self-facilitated by the district nurse or the team members involved. It is rarely planned or facilitated by someone with the skills or specialism to do so. As such, briefs in contemporary district nursing practice can be time-limited, unplanned and undocumented, with key learning points and actions unrecorded or often not taken forward. This can limit reflection, learning and practice development.

Think about:

How often are debriefs evaluated?

Do members of the group really have a chance, immediately after an incident, to reflect on what happened and explore their own feelings and role?

Other health professions have utilised the process of clinical supervision as a means to reflect, explore and be mindful about their practice in a small facilitated group environment. The next section of the chapter will explore clinical supervision and person-centred development (PCD) as an additional means of reflection and professional and personal development.

Clinical Supervision or Person-centred Development (PCD)?

Historical Perspective and Moving from Clinical Supervision towards PCD

Clinical supervision was introduced into clinical practice in the 1920s. The aim was to facilitate PCD. Clinical supervision can occur on a one-to-one basis or as a small group, being supervised by one supervisor to facilitate proceedings. Hence, there is a relationship between the supervisor and the person(s) involved. This partnership should be of equal status between all parties and should not reflect any type of management hierarchy. The primary focus should be on the needs of the supervisee(s), but the needs of facilitator(s) should not be negated. In some situations, the supervisors also need support and require a means to have their needs 'facilitated'.

> **Definition:**
>
> Elliott (2013, p. 174) defines clinical supervision as being 'about a supervisor facilitating supervisees to reflect on their past, present and future behaviour and its consequences'.

Purpose and Benefits

In many clinical areas, clinical supervision is embedded in practice. Many professionals find it an important part of their everyday work and rely on it in order to maintain their professional equilibrium, both physically and mentally. In other professions, the culture is not one of discussing, but of carrying on and doing. Elliott (2013, p. 169) suggests that clinical supervision should be part of all healthcare organisations and should be happening as a matter of course. It should be available to all, irrespective of their appointment, role or status. The focus should definitely not be on corporate or management objectives.

However, the organisation will also benefit, as supervisees will have more self-awareness and insight into their own practice. They may have more understanding of their accountability and potential to be fallible. For the organisation, this may translate into reducing adverse incidents involving patients, and staff taking greater professional accountability and responsibility for their own practice. More importantly, the patient should benefit from higher-quality care and a safer journey.

All writers on this subject (Cassedy 2010; Elliott 2013) warn of the danger of clinical supervision being facilitated by a line manager, where the process will then have managerial connotations. This is not how clinical supervision should be facilitated.

Key Features and Optimising Usefulness in Structure and Process

The following bullet points reflect the research of Winstanley and White (2003, p. 25), who found that clinical supervision is most effective, positive and productive if it includes the following elements:

♦ Sessions around 60 minutes in length
♦ At least monthly sessions (if not more frequent)
♦ Group sessions rather than one-to-one
♦ Conducted away from the participants' workplace
♦ Supervisor selected by the participants rather than allocated to the role.

The role of supervisor should: encourage supervisees to challenge their own attitudes, values and beliefs; encourage supervisees to push the limits of their thinking and to question their own work-based activities and those of others in a professional manner. The clinical supervision process may have multiple benefits for individuals, which are summarised below:

♦ Reduction in stress levels, less risk of burnout and reduction in emotional stress
♦ Improved self-awareness
♦ Improved self-esteem
♦ Improved confidence
♦ Helping the person to reflect and think about their practice
♦ Feeling more supported and valued
♦ Improvement in the person's depth of knowledge and understanding
♦ Enhanced personal and professional development
♦ A greater sense of personal achievement and satisfaction at work
♦ More confidence and support when challenging the poor practice or behaviour of colleagues.

Care must be taken that the clinical supervision process does not become a means of staff surveillance and is not seen in this way (Cassedy 2010; Hawkins and Shohet 2012). For district nurses, clinical supervision may provide a means of support and practice discussion for what can be a lonely profession in some respects. However, as you can now appreciate, it is more than just a discussion about practice issues. The term 'clinical supervision' may provide a misleading understanding of the process, implying directing, controlling or watching over others. For many staff, clinical supervision has become imposed and prescriptive. Elliott (2013) argues that it is time to redefine the term and proposes the use of the term 'person-centred development'.

Person-centred Development (PCD)

Advocates of PCD are clear that it has a universal meaning, which cannot be misunderstood or manipulated by employers:

Person – the individual
Centred – a focal point
Development – personal and professional growth, progress and advancement

The process of 'PCD promotes personal and professional development. During the process it can also have a positive effect on the individual and can serve to facilitate physical, psychological and social wellbeing' (Elliott 2013, p. 184). The words chosen imply a biopsychosocial approach, where physical, psychological and social aspects are of the utmost importance.

Role of the Facilitator

The PCD process should not include management in any form and it is inappropriate for facilitation to be conducted by a line manager or anyone holding a management position, especially if that manager is likely to be in a position where they may have a conflict of interest. Individuals should be able to choose their facilitator. If a new member of staff joins the organisation, the staff member should be supported if (at a later date) they decide they do not want the facilitator originally allocated to them.

The factors identified in Table 12.2 will impact upon the PCD session. The outcome of a PCD session will therefore depend upon the facilitator's understanding of and ability to integrate and apply the factors in order to achieve positive outcomes for the session. Some of the factors identified are things that we would assume are a given, but it is important for the facilitator to ensure that each of these are given equal importance and thought.

Role of the Participant

Individuals should be offered PCD, but should not be forced to take part. The facts of how the PCD approach will be facilitated should be given, so that individuals can make an informed decision and not be coerced. It is hoped that individuals will experience the benefit of PCD and value it as an option available to them. Also, the PCD process breeds its own success, as participants find it valuable and a source of motivation to continue.

As a relatively new approach, PCD was initiated by Engle (1980) and developed by Ogden (2012), who identifies factors that can inform and impact on the PCD relationship of the facilitator and the participant, as identified in Table 12.2. Many of the factors identified as important are directly relevant to district nurses and other healthcare workers.

Consideration should be given to the majority of the factors in Table 12.2. The facilitator should be prepared to manage potentially difficult situations. For example, if a participant is fatigued, they are more likely to misinterpret or miscommunicate what is being said or the style of communication, whether verbal or non-verbal. Thus, a facilitator needs to be prepared to resolve any such miscommunication. The ethos behind PCD is more holistic in nature and more of a partnership between the facilitator and the individual, and between the participants within the group.

Table 12.2 – Factors that can inform and impact the PCD relationship

Physical aspects	Time of day
	Workload
	Identifying a dedicated time for PCD to occur, and it not being routinely cancelled
	Physical fatigue
	Hunger/thirst

Table 12.2 – Factors that can inform and impact the PCD relationship (*continued*)

	Comfort – seating, body space
	Environment – room, temperature, lighting, ventilation
	Linking PCD sessions to duty rotas
	Flexible working
Psychological aspects	Degree of stress/anxiety
	Sense of personal safety
	Attitudes
	Freedom of choice
	Sense of acceptance into the group
	Sense of belonging
	Freedom from ridicule
	Feeling valued
	Past experience of group sessions
	Mood
	Motivation
	Communication – verbal, non-verbal
	Promotion of self-esteem
Social aspects	Confidentiality
	Establishing agreed-upon ground rules of the group
	Provision of education aimed at PCD and dissemination of information to all employees
	Sense of equality
	Facilitation, not dictation
	Self-expression
	Personal gain
	Maintaining dignity
	Receiving appropriate information

The success of PCD can also be affected by the culture, age and gender of the individuals present at the session. The attitude of participants will affect the success of the approach, as will their understanding of the purpose of the session. Participants must be assured that their workload will be covered during PCD sessions. Participants who have a sense that they are needed back at work will understandably find it difficult to focus their attention during sessions.

Think about:

As district nurses working at an advanced level and as independent prescribers, maybe a fresh approach to providing yourselves with support in your new role is what is required.

PCD may provide you as a group of prescribers with a way forward to personal and professional development.

It is perfectly possible for each of you to take on the role of facilitator on a rotational basis and to discuss if this works for you all.

It may be pertinent for you to now consider your professional CPD requirements and review if the information included in this chapter may be useful for the CPD process.

Conclusion

The concept of reflection has been explored. This chapter has provided some useful and varied ideas to help the clinician develop their ability to reflect in a more meaningful way. Reflection is very much a personal aspect of professional practice, where one size will not fit all, and therefore this chapter has presented a mixture of approaches. Person-centred development has been explored, with some ideas on how this may be applied to district nursing prescribing practice.

Key Points of This Chapter

- Understanding the connotations and expectations of professional practice should contribute to your advanced prescribing practice.
- Reflection is an important part of both personal and professional development.
- Self-awareness, persistence and the willingness to be honest and open are the key to reflecting effectively.
- Various reflective models exist. These may be useful to provide structure and direction to the reflective process.

> ♦ Person-centred development is a more recent approach, designed to explore the biopsychosocial aspects of a professional's role, and may be more beneficial than clinical supervision.
> ♦ CPD is part of your role and responsibilities as a health professional.

References and Further Reading

Benner, P. (2000) *From Novice to Expert: Excellence and Power in Clinical Nursing Practice.* Upper Saddle River, NJ: Prentice Hall.

Bolton, G. (2005) *Reflective Practice: Writing and Professional Development.* 2nd edn. London: Sage.

Bolton, G. (2010) *Reflective Practice: Writing and Professional Development.* 3rd edn. London: Sage.

Bolton, G. and Delderfield, R. (2018) *Reflective Practice: Writing and Professional Development.* 4th edn. London: Sage.

Bulman, C. and Schutz, S. (eds) (2013) *Reflective Practice in Nursing.* 5th edn. Chichester: John Wiley & Sons.

Carper, B. (1978) Fundamental patterns of knowing in nursing. *Advances in Nursing Science* 1(1): 13–23.

Cassedy, P. (2010) *First Steps in Clinical Supervision: A Guide for Healthcare Professionals.* Maidenhead: Open University Press/McGraw-Hill.

Council of Wales Deanery (2018) CPD for General Practitioners. Available at: https://gpcpd.walesdeanery.org/index.php/reflecting-on-prescribing (last accessed 13 August 2019).

Downie, J. (1989) *Professional Judgement: The Getting of Judgement.* Milton Keynes: Open University Press.

Elliott, P. (2013) Moving from clinical supervision to person-centred development: A paradigm change. In M. Jasper, G. Mooney and M. Rosser (eds), *Professional Development, Reflection and Decision Making in Nursing and Healthcare.* 2nd edn. Chichester: Wiley Blackwell, pp. 168–203.

Engle, G. L. (1980) The clinical application of the biopsychosocial model. *American Journal of Psychiatry* 137: 525–544.

Gibbs, G. (1988) *Learning by Doing: A Guide to Teaching and Learning Methods.* Oxford: Further Education Unit, Oxford Polytechnic.

Hawkins, P. and Shohet, R. (2012) *Supervision in the Helping Professions.* 4th edn. Maidenhead: Open University Press/McGraw-Hill.

Jasper, M. (2008) Learning journals and diary keeping. In C. Bulman and S. Schutz (eds), *Reflective Practice in Nursing.* 4th edn. Chichester: John Wiley & Sons, pp. 163–188.

Jasper, M. (2013) *Beginning Reflective Practice.* 2nd edn. Cheltenham: Nelson Thornes.

Jasper, M. and Mooney, G. (2013) Reflective writing for professional development. In M. Jasper, G. Mooney and M. Rosser (eds), *Professional Development, Reflection and Decision Making in Nursing and Healthcare.* 2nd edn. Chichester: Wiley Blackwell, pp. 83–108.

Jasper, M. and Rosser, M. (2013) Practising as a professional. In M. Jasper, G. Mooney and M. Rosser (eds), *Professional Development, Reflection and Decision Making in Nursing and Healthcare*. 2nd edn. Chichester: Wiley Blackwell, pp. 204–240.

Johns, C. (1995) Framing learning through reflection within Carper's fundamental ways of knowing in nursing. *Journal of Advanced Nursing* 22: 226–234.

Johns, C. (2017) *Becoming a Reflective Practitioner*. 5th edn. Oxford: Wiley Blackwell.

Kolb, D. A. (1984) *Experiential Learning: Experience as the Source of Learning and Development*. Upper Saddle River, NJ: Prentice Hall.

Maybin, J., Charles, A. and Honeyman, M. (2016) *Understanding Quality in District Nursing*. London: The King's Fund.

Nursing and Midwifery Council (NMC) (2001) *Standards for Specialist Practice*. London: NMC.

Nursing and Midwifery Council (NMC) (2019) *Evaluation of Post-Registration Standards of Proficiency for Specialist Community Public Health Nurses and the Standards for Specialist Education and Practice Standards*. London: Blake Stevenson Ltd.

Nursing Times News Desk (2019) NMC highlights the importance of nurses' reflection on practice. Available at: https://www.nursingtimes.net/news/professional-regulation/nmc-highlights-importance-of-nurses-reflection-on-practice/7029394.article (last accessed 13 August 2019).

Ogden, J. (2012) *Health Psychology: A Textbook*. 5th edn. Maidenhead: Open University Press/McGraw-Hill.

Queen's Nursing Institute (2015) *The QNI/QNIS Voluntary Standards for District Nurse Education and Practice*. London: The QNI.

Queen's Nursing Institute and the Royal College of Nursing (2019) *Outstanding Models of District Nursing. A Joint Project Identifying What Makes an Outstanding District Nursing Service*. London: The QNI/RCN.

Ramsey, C. (2005) Narrating development: Professional practice emerging within stories. *Action Research* 3(3): 279–295.

Rolfe, G., Freshwater, D. and Jasper, M. (2001) *Critical Reflection for Nursing and the Helping Professions: A User's Guide*. 2nd edn. Basingstoke: Palgrave Macmillan.

Schön, D. A. (1983) *The Reflective Practitioner*. London: Temple Smith.

Schön, D. A. (1987) *Educating the Reflective Practitioner*. San Francisco, CA: Jossey-Bass.

Winstanley, J. and White, E. (2003) Clinical supervision models, measures and best practice. *Nurse Researcher* 10(4): 7–38.

Useful Websites

NHS Leadership Academy: www.leadershipacademy.nhs.uk.

Index